The Unique Triple A™ Safety Handbook

The Unique Triple A™ Safety Handbook

How To Defend Yourself Without A Fight

Diane A Robinson

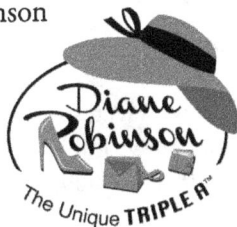

Printed in the United States of America.
First printing, 2015

ART, COVER DESIGNS:
Copyright © by: Janelle Carbajal

http:/www.YEAHNELL.COM
EDITING BY:
Ebook Editing Services

http:/www.ebookeditingservices.com
FORMATTING BY:
CreateSpace

http:/www.createspace.com
ISBN: 9780991509607
ISBN: 0991509609

Visit Diane At:
http://www.dianerobinsonauthor.com

Warning-Disclaimer

This book is designed as a **guide** to provide information on the three *Unique Triple A*™ strategies for self-defense: 1) to eliminate potential dangers from our lives by being more **ALERT** to surroundings, 2) to be more **AWARE** to recognize potential threats at the earliest possible stages, and 3) to **AVOID** potential dangers.

It is not the purpose of this handbook to be a substitute for proper training in self-defense and the martial arts. Every effort has been made to make this handbook as a **general basic guide only** and not as an ultimate source on the subjects or skills presented. Material presented is for information and entertainment only, and by reading further you accept any and all responsibility for any damage and risk, psychologically and/or physically to you and/or to someone else, that may result from the use or application of any information assimilated from this handbook. Anyone practicing the suggested skills or techniques presented in this handbook should be physically healthy enough to do so and understand how to use them.

You are urged to read all available material, learn as much as you wish about the covered subjects, and **tailor the information to your individual needs.** In consideration of reading this handbook **guide** and using its information, you waive all rights of damages against the author, publisher, printer, and distributors who shall neither have liability nor responsibility to any person or entity with respect to loss or damages caused, alleged to have been used, directly or indirectly, by the information within this handbook.

Please note most states contain laws in legal responsibility for use of any defense techniques or weapons against another person. An important phrase is that the victim must **believe** that bodily injury is about to be inflicted. Keep in mind that this handbook guide was not written for you to use to bully, cajole, threaten, or intimidate others, nor is the last word on self-defense, and that it is recommended, if you choose, that you seek proper instruction with a certified instructor who can observe and coach you on proper self-defense and offense techniques.

Aknowledgements

This book would not have been possible without the generous support of so many people who gave freely of their time. Success is all about believing in yourself. Mentors/coaches do make a significant difference in your life to blossom powerfully in learning and sharing. In alphabetical order:

Barbara Buck, Kate Conrad, Joanie Harmon, and Linda Pierce, my talented writing support/friendship group.

Christopher J. Lynch, *One-Eyed Jack* novels, for his workshops and insight. http://www.christopherjlynch.com

Ian Houghton, the ultimate coach of *Just Do It* books. Ian will never settle for less what one can be by getting you to your personal development.
http://www.ianhoughton.com

Janelle Carbajal, for creating awesome book covers and my brand logo. http://www.yeahnelle.com

Kate Stewart, for her professionalism, support, skillful editing, and patience.
http://www.ebookediting sevices.com

Nutschell A. Windsor, her staff and writing workshops.
http://www.cbw.la.org

My family for their love, patience and support.

God, because whatever glory comes from this endeavor in making a difference in people and communities belong to Him.

Each one of us has unlimited power lying within you to touch others and make a difference. You are all unlimited.

Visit Diane At:
http://www.dianerobinsonauthor.com

Table of Contents

Foreword

by Ian Houghton

Ian Houghton is the best-selling author of *The JFDI Way to Increasing Profits Through Outstanding Customer Service.* He is a leading authority on increasing profits through outstanding customer service and customer experience. Dubbed by one of the world's top business coaches (JT Foxx), as "The British Business Sensation" and "Master of Implementation," Ian is also an internationally-renowned speaker, business mentor, award-winning real estate entrepreneur, and coach.

Diane has been an outstanding student of mine by creating *The Unique Triple A™ Safety Handbook: How To Defend Yourself Without A Fight.* What makes this book so unique is Diane's own unique self-discovery journey into her senior years and on the way to producing this book for you. Diane pushed hard and overcame many obstacles due to her overwhelming passion she has for making the lives of others as safe as possible. Combining her 35+ years in the police force, and numerous years as a bodyguard to some of the world's top celebrities, she is able to combine these years of know-how into this simple, easy-to-use handbook and guide.

You now have the opportunity to learn from someone so caring and knowledgeable about the art of common sense in self-defense, you now can be prepared to defend with *The Unique Triple A™* should you ever need to.

Together, Diane and I finely tuned the direction of this book in order to give you maximum information the simplest possible way. You are about to discover some of the most powerful, proven, and most effective ways of using common sense in self-defense by one of the most experienced and knowledgeable people in the industry. If, and only if you take action, "Just Do It," and read this book, your knowledge will drastically increase.

Ian Houghton
Award-winning real estate entrepreneur, international speaker, business mentor, and best-selling author of *Just Do It.*
http://www.IanHoughton.com

Introduction

Dear Reader:

I want to thank you for purchasing my book. I am honored to share my mission with you. This is not a book how to use weapons or martial arts, as you can find those through bookstores or self-defense studios. My book is for men, women, children, and seniors of all ages who are concerned about crime and safety. Crime is not something we like to think about.

You are going to read three key words, **ALERT, AWARE, AVOID,** so many times in this book that they will be inscribed into your brain and mindset. Remember when you first started typing on the keyboard looking down at the keys? With practice, the subconscious mind memorized the keyboard until you no longer looked down. That repeated process programmed a subconscious mindset for you to type away without looking at those keys. Much in the same way, these daily readings from *The Unique Triple A™ Safety Handbook: How To Defend Yourself Without A Fight* and its three principles, **ALERT, AWARE, AVOID** can be programmed into your subconscious mind.

By investing in *The Unique Triple A™* three principles, you have empowered and benefited yourself and others in your community.

1. **ALERT**
2. **AWARE**
3. **AVOID**

How This Guide Will Work For You

The Unique Triple A™ will guide you to be **ALERT** to your surroundings, to be **AWARE** to recognize potential dangerous situations, and to **AVOID** them.

How?

About the Cover:

First, **BEFORE** you start this book, take a good observation of the book cover, then take the **Book Cover Observation Test** under QUESTIONS: A Reading Group Guide. Suggested answers are provided. The cover design illustrates crimes of opportunity in order to understand the *Unique Triple A*™ principles. How well did you do with the **Book Cover Observation Test**?

How?

About the Logo:

Second, take a look at my brand logo to understand why, etc.

HAT: Large brim hats obstruct views to be **ALERT** of areas/persons.

PURSE: AVOID fighting for purse and a tug of war with assailant.

SHOE: Be **AWARE** if you can run in high heels to escape safely.

WALLET: Be **ALERT** wallets are easy targets for pickpocketing.

The Unique Triple A™ *Safety Handbook: How To Defend Yourself Without A Fight* is designed around my passionate purpose and mission to inspire educate, empower, and encourage others by raising **ALERTNESS, AWARENESS** to **AVOID** potential threats. I am blessed to have the gifts of knowledge and expertise from my law enforcement career to give back and make a difference to others and communities. Your purchase also goes towards helping you and others in your community.

Too many believe that martial arts requires great physical skills and athletic proficiency. Yet, preventative measures are easily learned, requires almost no athletic ability, and can be mastered by anyone at any age. Remember, even the best trained martial artist **AVOIDS** potential dangerous situations or put themselves in a dangerous situation.

I love this perpetual calendar handbook, and there is space on the pages for you to write your thoughts. I feel passionately blessed and so much appreciation to give back as you make an investment to enhance your life and others.

Now, are you passionate enough to be **ALERT, AWARE** and **AVOID** reducing chances of being a victim?

You are BRAVER than you believe, STRONGER than you seem, and SMARTER than you think.

Diane A. Robinson
May 2015

*"He has shown you what is good, and what
does the Lord require of you?"*

MICAH 6:8

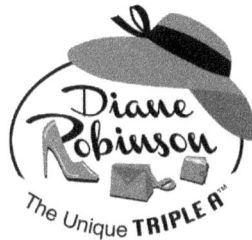

Diane Robinson

The Unique TRIPLE A™

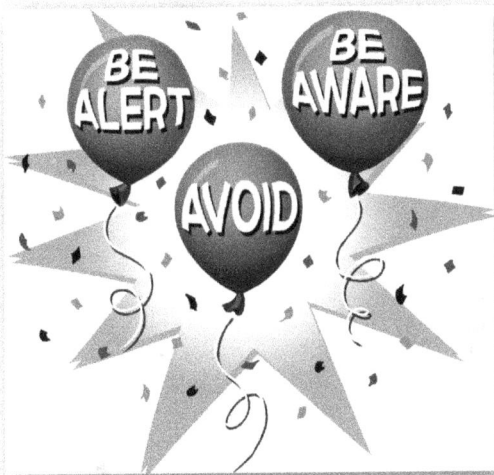

January

SAFETY RESOLUTIONS

———

New Beginnings

January 1

HAPPY NEW YEAR!

Are your New Year resolutions each year realistic enough to stick with them? Do you consider home and workplace safety? What about personal safety? January is a month of new beginnings filled with 31 brief, but basic safety resolutions.

Tradition dictates that every 365 days, one should attempt to kick bad habits and start the New Year with new resolutions. The New Year brings great hopes for change, growth and presents the perfect time to set some resolutions that can help make your life more positive, productive and enjoyable. Start the New Year and improve your personal safety.

WHEREAS, I commit to being responsible for my own actions and how they impact risk factors to the safety of family and friends.
*WHEREAS, I will begin to be **ALERT, AWARE** and **AVOID** dangerous risks.*
WHEREAS, I will try to get at least 6 hours of sleep.
WHEREAS, I will try to exercise ___ a week.

_____   _____

Signature   Date

January 2

The Unique Triple A™ strategies are practical and make common sense as an intelligent approach to safety in all areas of our lives, including health and fitness.

1. Be **ALERT** to your surroundings.
2. Be **AWARE** to recognize, and
3. **AVOID** potential dangers.

It's about changing your mindset and bad habit behaviors.

Today's Exercise...

Sit down, relax, gather your thoughts and write out some areas of yourself, home, and workplace that need safety and personal improvement, because tomorrow is the first of your daily *The Unique Triple A*™ safety practices.

January 3

In this handbook you are provided monthly crime prevention topics followed by daily affirmations that offer guidance and support to help stay safe. These 365 readings help you to re-member, each day, to stay focused and centered on new safety beginnings throughout the year, supported by *The Unique Triple A*™ safety strategies, **ALERT, AWARE, AVOID,** with added space for your comments and thoughts.

Yes, everything from high-tech communication devices to smart cards do make our lives safer and more secure.

Yet, when you did yesterday's exercise to write out the safety weaknesses in your personal life, home, and workplace, were you any safer or secure? What did you find?

"Good judgment comes from experience,
and experience, well, that comes
from poor judgment."
~ ANONYMOUS

January 4
ALCOHOL AND DRUGS

AVOID throwing caution to the wind by being careless and irresponsible to the safety of yourself and others throughout the year. As holidays, celebrations, and parties occur throughout the year, remember the following:

- **AVOID** drinking, drugs, and driving.
- Know your safe limits.
- Your consequences impact you, your family, friends, workplace, and community.
- **AVOID** those who are drunk and disorderly.
- Drinking too much alcohol can have lethal affects. Be responsible.
- **AVOID** legal risks of drug/alcohol risk crimes.

January 5

Monitor Your Alcohol Intake...

Use as a reference only and should not be relied upon to determine whether you are capable of operating a motor vehicle. Always keep in mind that there are a number of variables that can influence whether you are legally qualified to drive.

DRINK CHART GUIDE

(a guide - not a guarantee)

YOUR WEIGHT	NUMBER OF DRINKS (over a two-hour period) 1-1/4 ozs. 80 proof liquor, 12 oz. can of beer or 4 ozs. of wine.							
90 to 109	1	2	3	4	5	6	7	8
110 to 129	1	2	3	4	5	6	7	8
130 to 149	1	2	3	4	5	6	7	8
150 to 169	1	2	3	4	5	6	7	8
170 to 189	1	2	3	4	5	6	7	8
190 to 209	1	2	3	4	5	6	7	8
210 to 229	1	2	3	4	5	6	7	8
230 & UP	1	2	3	4	5	6	7	8

☐ (.01% - .04%) May be DUI ☐ (.05% - .07%) Likely DUI ☐ (.08% - UP) Definitely DUI

BLOOD ALCOHOL LEVELS

One drink is considered:

(1) 12 fl oz beer

(1) 5 fl oz glass of wine

(1) 1.5 fl oz shot of hard liquor

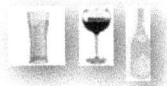

Source: http://www.drunkdriving.org/blood_alcohol_levels.html

January 6

Party Tips Throughout The Year...

- When attending a party, use a different cup or colored glass for your personal use.
- It will aide you to be **ALERT** and **AWARE** if someone switched your drink or you picked up the wrong drink.
- **AVOID** leaving your drink unattended and **AVOID** walking away from your drink for the dance floor, restroom. Finish the drink, throw it away, or take it with you.
- **AVOID** accepting open drinks from others who you do not know or trust.
- **AVOID** sharing beverages with others.
- **AVOID** becoming intoxicated.

January 7

- Be **AWARE** of your surroundings at all times.
- Criminals often confront people who are distracted or drunk.
- Be **ALERT** to your condition and **AWARE** that drugs can be slipped into your unattended drink.
- **AVOID** drinking alcoholic beverages without eating first.
- Eat high protein foods that stay in the stomach longer.
- They also slow the absorption of alcohol into your system.
- Drink responsibly.
- Party with responsible friends.
- Enjoy the upcoming Chinese New Year safely.

January 8

- Go to parties, clubs, and bars with a group of friends and agree beforehand to leave together. **AVOID** being separated from your friends.
- Arrange a designated meeting place and exchange cell phone numbers in case you become separated.
- **AVOID** taking off alone without telling your friends, or group you are with, where you will be and the person's information.
- If you meet someone, arrange another time during the day to meet in a public place and **AVOID** giving out your personal information.
- Be **ALERT** and **AWARE** of "burner phones" (see GLOSSARY), that can be purchased and used when you want to **AVOID** giving out a personal phone number.
- **AVOID** leaving iPads and phones unattended for thieves. Be **AWARE** if your phone has a GPS or other program on it to track the phone or you.

January 9

- **AVOID** wearing expensive or fancy jewelry, or bringing more valuables than you need, which puts you and your values at risk.
- You may want attention, but not the wrong attraction.
- Dress casually and comfortably.
- If you do carry cash, divide it between your pockets, purse, and wallet.
- **AVOID** displaying large sums of cash. Only carry the items that you are going to need for going out, such as a credit card and amount of cash needed.
- **AVOID** carrying all your checks or checkbook.

January 10

Be ALERT And AWARE To The Following Facts...

Though you may not be the person using alcohol or drugs, you can certainly be a victim of an alcohol or drug-related crime.

- Each year more than 600,000 students between the ages of 18 and 24 are assaulted by another student who has been drinking.
- 95 percent of all violent crime on college campuses involves the use of alcohol by the assailant, victim, or both.
- Every day 36 people die, and approximately 700 are injured, in motor vehicle crashes that involve an alcohol-impaired driver. Drinking and drugged driving is the number one cause of death, injury, and disability of young people under the age of 21.

Source: National Crime Prevention Council, Alcohol, Drugs and Crime (NCADD). http://www.ncadd.org

January 11

DRIVING

- **AVOID** drinking, drugs, and driving.
- Check with your community for any organizational ride programs.
- Be **ALERT** to several alternatives if unable to drive. Stay at a local hotel, be with friends who watch out for each other, have a non-drinker friend as a designated driver in your group of friends, or call a cab.
- Be **AWARE** if out of town and staying at a hotel to make arrangements with your hotel, or a cab company, to pick you up at the designated location away from the hotel.

January 12

<u>Be A Proactive Driver, Make Safety Resolutions</u>...

*WHEREAS, I will **AVOID** the use of a cell phone behind the wheel of a car, unless in case of an emergency.*

*WHEREAS, I will be **ALERT** to drive the speed limit (speeding is a factor in about one-third of all fatal crashes).*

WHEREAS, I will always buckle up and ensure my passengers will do the same.

WHEREAS, I will always make a full stop at stop signs and look all ways before pulling forward safely.

WHEREAS, I will be more fuel efficient by keeping tires properly inflated, obeying speed limits, and routine vehicle maintenance.

_____   _____
Signature   Date

January 13

WHEREAS, I will actively pay attention to cars in front of, and behind me.

*WHEREAS, I will **AVOID** being near swerving cars.*

WHEREAS, I will call police if there is a possible drunk driver.

WHEREAS, I will cross carefully when signal lights turn green.

*WHEREAS, I will be **AWARE** my cell phone is fully charged.*

*WHEREAS, I will be **ALERT** and **AWARE** that car is in good mechanical order and filled with gas.*

*WHEREAS, I will **AVOID** going home if being followed and drive to the nearest well-lit or populated area.*

WHEREAS, I will know where emergency locations are in area, such as police, fire, hospitals, and gas stations.

_____   _____

Signature   Date

January 14

<u>**When Leaving A Party, Restaurant, Gym, Home...**</u>

- **AVOID** waiting until you get to your car to look for your keys.
- Be **ALERT** and have your keys in your hand before you get to the door.
- Keys, placed in-between fingers, are one of the offensive weapons as described under WEAPONS.
- Be **AWARE** of the panic alarm button on your key fob to use when in danger.
- Be **AWARE** of your surroundings before approaching your car.
- Be **ALERT** to look around, under, and inside your car before entering.

January 15

HOSTESS WITH THE MOSTESS

As a host, be **AWARE** that your resolutions should include children when you host parties, holidays, or big family get-togethers in your home.

- Be **AWARE** to make the alcoholic and non-alcoholic punch different colors in different bowls.
- Use different color cups or glasses to serve alcoholic and nonalcoholic drinks, especially if there are underage guests in attendance.
- Keep all stairways closed off to toddlers to **AVOID** unwanted falls and children going into areas that are not child friendly, such as kitchens and bathrooms.

January 16

As a host, be **AWARE** that your resolutions should include pets when you host parties, holidays, or big family get-togethers in your home, as they become excited or nervous when brought together in these events.

- Unless you know your pets, **AVOID** guests and children from handling your pets, or keep pets in a different room if not outside.
- Loud noises can confuse and irritate pets.
- Be sure they are secured, have food and water.
- Keep their favorite toys nearby for comfort and play.

January 17

ATHLETIC, GYM RESOLUTIONS

*WHEREAS, I will be **ALERT** and **AWARE** that virtually any article left in plain view, unattended, or unlocked is apt to be stolen.*

*WHEREAS, I will **AVOID** leaving keys unattended.*

WHEREAS, I will use a lock on the gym locker.

WHEREAS, I will leave personal items of value at home.

*WHEREAS, I will be **AWARE** to look for escape routes, or which streets to use when jogging.*

*WHEREAS, I will be **AWARE** of surroundings in and outside the gym/areas when exiting and returning to car.*

WHEREAS, I will take photos and/or keep a written record (descriptions, serial numbers) of valuables that can aid in a stolen property report.

_____   _____

Signature   Date

January 18

CYBER SAFETY

- Be **ALERT** and always keep passwords private and change them often.
- Be **ALERT** and **AWARE** of making passwords safer without keyboard strokes as follows:
- Write out a short title from a movie, poem, song, phrase, then take the first letter of each word (add numbers, capitals, etc.), to make a password and "bury" in a word document (be sure document is saved in a flash drive, not hard drive). Copy and paste onto log in password box to **AVOID** hacking, recording, or tracking of keyboard strokes for criminal acts.
- **AVOID** giving out personal information and only order things online from websites safely used before.
- **AVOID** opening e-mails, or visiting websites, that don't seem trustworthy and may contain a virus or malware that may harm computer.

January 19

DINING OUT

When dining, in addition to your napkin, the only place your purse should be, is securely on your lap. Be **ALERT** that you are **AWARE** that your purse or travel handbag can never be out of your view.

- Victims of purse snatches are too deeply involved in the dining and socializing process to be **AWARE** of their personal belongings and often **AVOID** paying attention to their belongings.
- **AVOID** leaving your purse on the back of your chair, on the floor, or by your side.
- Be **AWARE** your purse is zipped and closed at all times.
- **AVOID** and be **ALERT** to tables and chairs that are placed closely together.

January 20

PARKING SAFETY RESOLUTIONS

*WHEREAS, I will **AVOID** parking in isolated and poorly lit areas.*

*WHEREAS, I will make a note where parked to **AVOID** wandering around and attract a suspect.*

*WHEREAS, I will be **AWARE** to run errands and shop early with the buddy system, or park as close to the stores as possible.*

*WHEREAS, I will **AVOID** waiting until getting to the car to look for keys.*

*WHEREAS, I will be **ALERT** that my keys are placed in-between fingers as a defense weapon.*

*WHEREAS, I will be **AWARE** of the use of the panic alarm button on my key fob.*

*WHEREAS, I will be **AWARE** of surroundings and be **ALERT** to look around, under, and inside car before approaching and entering.*

WHEREAS, I will immediately place all items in car, lock all doors after entering, and immediately leave.

WHEREAS, I will sort packages later after safely driving off.

_____   _____

Signature   Date

January 21

Sound The Alarm...

- Be **ALERT** to carry keys in the offensive position (between fingers), while walking to your car in a parking lot.
- Be **AWARE** of the panic button on your car fob. If you feel you are in danger near your car, press the button to activate the car's security alarm system to gain attention for help.
- Be **AWARE** to keep your car keys next to your bed when you retire for the evening.
- If you think someone is attempting to break into your home, first call the police, go to safety, and press the panic alarm button on your car key remote to sound your car's security alarm system. **AVOID** staying in house.
- Always remember the car alarm or horn will continue until either the battery runs down or until you reset it with the button on the key fob.

January 22

PURSE SAFETY

- Be **ALERT** and **AWARE** to always keep a secure hold on purse and wallet.
- Be a safety fashionista. Many stores sell very nice strapless purses that can be worn around the waist or wrist, rather than straps that can forcibly be pulled away from in an attack.
- **AVOID** leaving personal property (computers, cell phones, backpacks, purses) unattended in classrooms, dressing rooms, grocery carts, public restrooms, and under theater seats.
- **AVOID** placing purse atop the car when placing items inside car. It only takes a second for a thief to grab it.

January 23

- Carry as little paper currency as possible and only the credit cards and checks needed for the day.
- Carry keys, glasses, or medication separately from purse. If a purse is taken this helps **AVOID** a health issue and loss of transportation. Keys and ID are information to the thief to gain entry to home (change locks immediately), and identify theft.
- **AVOID** being a creature of bad habits.
- **AVOID** struggling for purse that can cause a fall and extreme physical injury to accomplish the criminal act.
- **AVOID** carrying pin numbers, account numbers, or any safe combination numbers.
- Be **AWARE** that unsnapping a top snap on a small clutch purse and turning it upside down allows the contents to spill out and distract the thief that may allow time to run **AWAY** from assailant for help.

January 24

OUT AND ABOUT

- Be **AWARE** and try to wear comfortable clothes and shoes.
- Be **AWARE** to have the aura of a confident person with purpose. Be **AWARE, ALERT,** and **AVOID** uncomfortable situations or persons.
- Be **ALERT** and **AWARE** of your surroundings at all times.
- **AVOID** distractions, such as talking on cell phone or listening to music with earphones while walking or jogging. Distractions decease **AWARENESS**.
- **AVOID** talking to, or be distracted by street solicitors.
- Hold personal items, such as a purse, close and tight to your body.
- If you feel uncomfortable, go to the nearest opened store or well-populated area.
- Be **AWARE** and **ALERT** where local 24-hour emergency agencies (police, fire, hospital), and other 24-hour stores are located when needing assistance.

January 25

REALTOR SAFETY & SECURITY TIPS

The number of assaults against real estate professionals is on the rise and deadly. The Bureau of Labor Statistics reported 250,000 assaults (10 each hour), and over 150 fatal injuries nationwide. REALTORS® are targeted because they are crimes of opportunity, such as hosting open houses and visiting vacant properties.

Be ALERT, AWARE, AVOID

- Properly ID and pre-qualify at first meeting.
- First time clients should be required to send in a copy of their driver's license and full contact details.
- Arrange first meeting either at office or **PUBLIC PLACE**.
- Always let your office know where you are going and what client(s) in your file.
- Use the buddy system. Bring a co-worker with you, especially if you are a lone female and in vacant houses.
- Arrive at location at least 15 minutes early **BEFORE** opening to public.

Source: Bureau of Labor Statistics. http://www.bls.gov

January 26

REALTOR SAFETY & SECURITY TIPS

- Be **ALERT** to check garage area, signs of forced entry or open doors/windows **BEFORE** you enter. If so, leave, call police.

- When entering, be **AWARE** and **ALERT** to look for exits and "danger" areas, such as back yard, garage. Be **ALERT** to have a code system or color that can let office know you may need help. Example: Yellow can mean you would like someone to meet you at the next location ("look in the yellow folder...") Red for immediate assistance

- When giving tours of the home, be **ALERT** to stay **OUTSIDE** of the rooms. **NEVER** go in a room if you are a lone female. Let them enter first. Stay at the doorway to answer questions. When showing a home to more than one person, be **AWARE** they stay together.

- Be **AWARE** and **ALERT** how you dress.

- **AVOID** wearing expensive jewelry and shoes that hinder getting away.

- Carry a well-charged phone (programmed to 9-1-1).

- **APPS FOR PHONE**: Agents Armor; Watch Over Me.

January 27

Survey Says...

A do-it yourself security check home assessment.

YES NO FIX

EXTERIOR

O   O   O   Are you using decorative rock or stones around the perimeter?

O   O   O   Are gates properly locked and secured?

O   O   O   Are house numbers visible on home and curb for emergency personnel?

O   O   O   Are bikes, lawn mowers, hoses, locked up when not in use?

WINDOWS

O   O   O   Are they kept closed and secured when away?

O   O   O   Are they open, but secured with appropriate anti-theft tools, when at home?

O   O   O   Are window air conditioners anchored and secured to prevent removal from outside?

NEIGHBORHOOD

O   O   O   Do you know or communicate with neighbors living on both sides of your home?

O   O   O   Is there an ACTIVE Neighborhood Watch program on your street?

January 28

APARTMENT SECURITY

- Be **ALERT** and **AWARE** of security issues when renting an apartment or condo.
- Be **ALERT** to conduct an outside perimeter and security checks on doors, windows before you make a decision to rent or lease the best you can find. A wooden frame door can be easily kicked to force entry.
- Apartment managers should use solid core doors and high quality Grade 1 or Grade 2 deadbolt locks on exterior doors that will resist twisting, prying, and lock-picking attempts.
- Always check with landlord before you install better locks. Be **AWARE** you may be given permission, but unless you can compromise on sharing security expenses, the landlord gains your safety installments as a better unit to rent out at a possible price increase when you leave.

January 29

- Be **ALERT** and **AWARE** of workplace safety and help enhance safety where I work.
- Be **ALERT** and **AWARE** if your workplace has a Workplace Violence Prevention Program and Sexual Assault Program. If not, inquire from law enforcement how to coordinate with management to implement a policy.
- Be **AWARE** a workplace can implement a sign-in ledger, guest pass badges, and be escorted by the person they are visiting to the location, and then escorted back to front desk or exit door.
- Follow the same caution with deliveries and pickups with identity checked.
- Be **ALERT** to keep purse, wallet, keys, or other valuables locked in a drawer or closet.
- Report any broken or flickering lights, dimly lit corridors, broken windows, and doors that don't lock properly.

January 30

- Immediately report signs of potential violence of a fellow employee to the appropriate person. Immediately report any incidents of sexual harassment.

- Know company emergency plans, and keep emergency supplies (flashlight, walking shoes, water bottle, nonperishable food), in a locked desk drawer.

- **AVOID** staying late or alone in the office.

- Create a buddy system for walking to parking area or ask a security guard to be an escort, if applicable.

- Be **ALERT** and **AWARE** of anyone making a delivery to your home office, and be properly identified before you open the door, if you have a home business.

- Install door viewer security products, such as a peephole for home.

January 31

An Ounce Of Prevention Is Worth A Pound Of Cure...

- Take the initiative to manage your overall safety and health. Help others, family, friends, and loved ones to make safety resolutions as well. Support each other.
- Incorporate *The Unique Triple A*™ safety tips and good health into your everyday routines and help make crime prevention and staying healthy a regular part of your daily life.
- Be **ALERT** not to make a resolution to try out something risky and dangerous you haven't prepared safely for, like parachuting, mountain climbing. **AVOID** putting yourself in an unsafe situation.
- Keep track of your blood pressure, cholesterol level, blood sugar, and schedule physical exams with your doctor. Eat healthy with fruits, vegetables, and plenty of water (see HEALTH RECORD SUMMARY).

BONUS SAFETY TIP

How are you prepared if first emergency responders can't get to you? September is National Preparedness Month, sponsored by the Federal Emergency Management Agency (FEMA), to educate, empower, and prepare you for emergencies and disasters. Take action before September and prepare emergency kits for car, home, and office, and create a family emergency plan.

A Brief Basic Disaster Supply Kit (at least 3 days)...

- One gallon of water per person per day
- Battery-powered or hand-crank radio, flashlight and extra batteries.

A Brief Fire Hazard Safety Checklist...

- Create a defensible space by removing perimeter flammable vegetation and replace with fire-resistance vegetation.
- Cover outside unscreened vents and clean out open eaves, rain gutters.

To find out more, refer to your local fire department, American Red Cross, and FEMA web sites.

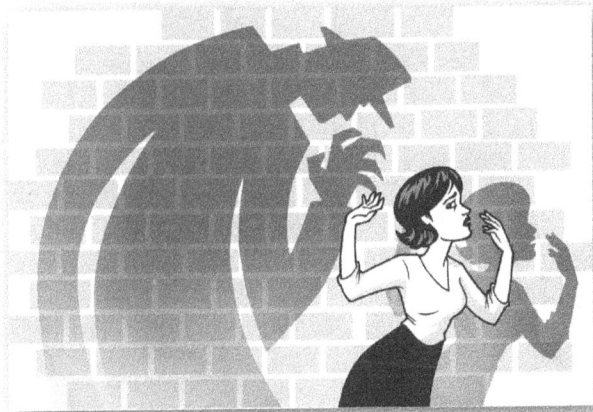

February

THE PRESIDENTIAL TREATMENT

Stalking

February 1

WHAT IS STALKING?

Stalking is a pattern of repeated and unwanted attention, harassment, contact, or any other course of tconduct directed to a specific person that would cause a reasonable person to feel fear. Stalking can include:

- Repeated, unwanted, intrusive, and frightening communications from the perpetrator by phone, mail, and/or e-mail.
- Sending unsolicited/unwanted letters or e-mails.
- Repeatedly leaving or sending victim unwanted items, presents, or flowers.
- Following or lying in wait for the victim at places such as home, school, work, or recreation places.
- Making direct or indirect threats to harm the victim, the victim's children, relatives, friends, or pets.
- Damaging or threatening to damage the victim's property.
- Harassing victim through the internet.

February 2

- Posting information or spreading rumors about the victim on the internet, in a public place, or by word of mouth.
- Obtaining personal information about the victim by accessing public records, using internet search services, hiring private investigators, going through the victim's garbage, following the victim, contacting victim's friends, family, work, or neighbors.

NOTE:

According to the latest Department of Justice figures, 6 million people are stalked each year in the United States, and social media is the number 1 reason such figures rose dramatically in the past decade.

Source: http://www.bjs.gov/index.cfm?ty=pbdetail&iid=1211
Source: Stalking Resource Center, National Center for Victims of Crime

February 3

BE YOUR OWN BODYGUARD

Bodyguards protect a person or persons, usually public, wealthy, politically important figures, from danger and responsible for their safety. Help protect yourself from danger. Why increase our chances of being victimized when you can do something?

- Wear common sense shoes and clothing that allow you freedom of movement.
- Did you ever see a bodyguard or president in high heels or skin-tight clothing?
- Practice makes perfect until it becomes natural to you.
- **AVOID** distractions, such as headgear for music, cell phones, or wide-brimmed hats that distract your senses for sight and hearing.
- Walk with assurance and confidence.
- Walk at a steady pace. Shoulders back, stand erect, head high, look around.
- Be **ALERT** and **AWARE** of your surroundings at all times.

February 4

- Keep your car secure. Keep doors locked at all times. Don't leave it running as you run a quick errand.
- **AVOID** aggressive drivers and road rage. **AVOID** playing games. Report to police and give vehicle license plate number and driver description.
- Some people who frequent bars like to drink and can become threatening, rude or aggressively drunk.
- If you find yourself in a situation at a bar or nightclub where a person is grabbing at you, **ALERT** the bartender and let them handle the situation.
- If you feel uncomfortable by the "look" of the crowd, walk out and find another nightclub destination. **AVOID** giving in to peer pressure to stay.
- Take only what you need, such as amount of money, credit card and identification card.

February 5

BODYGUARDS AND RELATIONSHIPS

- Consider your relationship with your partner or other social relationships.
- Be **AWARE** and **AVOID** triggers, which are any verbal or nonverbal behaviors that may result in anger or other negative emotional reactions that can harm you physically or mentally.
- Keep tabs on the health of your relationships and signs of domestic abuse.
- The only person who can guard you is yourself.

Today's Exercise...

How would you prepare your daily schedule or activities with safety, **ALERTNESS, AVOIDNESS,** and **AWARENESS** in mind?

February 6

BE STREET SMART

- Should you feel that you are being followed by another car, make several turns down active streets.
- Be **AWARE** if you are being followed, drive to the nearest well-lit or populated location, such as hospitals, gas stations, open stores, malls, fire and police buildings.

February 7

BE PEDESTRIAN SMART

- Be **ALERT** and **AWARE** that displaying expensive jewelry can be attractive to any opportunist thief.
- If you must wear high heels, also carry portable, soft slippers in purse.
- Be **ALERT** if a motorist or pedestrian bothers you while you are walking. Walk into a store or reverse your direction, or walk across the street to the other side safely.
- Secure your belongings and use keys as an offensive weapon by placing individual keys between fingers. Prepare to be in the Orange Zone and remain in this high state of **ALERTNESS** until you have quickly departed the area to safety (see COLOR CODES).
- Walk confidently while being **ALERT** and **AWARE**.
- You can always stop, turn around, and yell at the person to go away as you call the police. Keep cell phone in hand.

February 8

JOG, RUN, WALK, EXERCISE

- **AVOID** doing these activities alone, or in areas not well lit, unpopulated, or with numerous hiding places, such as shrubbery, alleys, or short cuts.

- **AVOID** taking short cuts and familiarize yourself with the area before heading out.

- VIP bodyguards know the beaten, well-traveled path is the better path. Even the president jogs with his security personnel.

- Many people like to listen to music while jogging, but be **AWARE** that it may prevent you from hearing the approach of persons, vehicles, or any other type of potential danger.

- **AVOID** using headphones or cell phones as the distraction may prevent you from being **ALERT** and **AWARE** of your surroundings, and **distract** your hearing, and sight. Only the president's bodyguards can get away with headgear.

- Wear bright colors. This will make you more visible to people and cars around you.

February 9

- Be **AWARE** not to carry valuables.
- **AVOID** displaying any jewelry. Just be **AWARE** that even cheap jewelry that appears expensive can be attractive to an opportunist thief.
- Select the proper type of shoes.
- **AVOID** injuries when jogging. Consult your doctor to evaluate your condition and offer advice. Warm up before you start to reduce the chance of muscle-pulls and strains.
- Be **ALERT** how your body feels after your physical activity. Aches and pains are not uncommon so stretch out again. However, be **AWARE** if sharp pains continue hours later which may be indicative of an injury. Consult medical advice.
- Always run against the flow of traffic. Roads with lower speed limits tend to be safer.
- Pick places where there's a wide shoulder. If there's a sidewalk, you're definitely better off on a sidewalk.

February 10

PUBLIC LISTINGS

- For phone directory listings, use first name initial with your last name and no street address.
- **AVOID** using your full name and address.
- Unlisted phone numbers are better.
- For mailboxes, use last name only. **AVOID** using your first name.
- For checks, driver's license, and registration, use first initial with your last name. Use a P.O. Box as address.

February 11

- Increase **AWARENESS** of risks and threats.
- Make time to master daily affirmations.
- Stay **AWARE**, focused, and stay safe.
- Use the best strategies in order to maintain resolutions and commitments for safety.
- Write out some strategy actions and learn ways to **AVOID** potentially unsafe situations and persons.

In life, most people know what to do, but few actually do what they know. Knowing is not enough.

February 12

CELLPHONE AND EMERGENCIES

- Does your smartphone have a mobile personal security system that uses GPS technology to instantly connect for help or a tracking system to find you?
- Below write your emergency numbers for hospital, doctor, child's school.

February 13

Abraham Lincoln (February 12, 1809 – April 15, 1865), was the 16th President of the United States, serving from March 1861 until his assassination in April 1865.

GOT A RED PHONE, TOO?

- When recording an outgoing message: **AVOID** leaving your name, phone number, or that you are not at home, on vacation.
- Another option is purchasing pre-recorded messages. Some choices include comedy and celebrity voices.
- If you are a female living alone, get a male friend to record messages using "we." "We ask you to leave a message," or "We will get back…"
- Even the president uses messages.
- Write out a sample for your message below.

"If it's the Psychic Network why do they need a phone number?"

~ ROBIN WILLIAMS

February 14

- Be the present to yourself. Give the gift of love to yourself. Remind yourself that you are worth loving. Always believe in yourself. Be the confident, optimistic you.

- Loving yourself is mainly having self-respect, the only dependable way to create love in your own life. You will mentally and physically take better care of yourself.

- Keep a journal. Write about your experiences, good and bad. When you write down good experiences, allow yourself to feel those feelings.

- Express yourself, perhaps in a diary, or through short stories. You can also do creative tasks, like painting or music.

- Define yourself by your efforts, not just your accomplishments.

- Practice meditation for 10 or 15 minutes a day to quiet your mind. Be **AWARE** of breathing air into your lungs, being in the moment, and not focusing on anything in the moment except air in and air out. It will help you love yourself and others more.

February 15

Today's Exercise...

I embrace negatives into positives.
I believe in myself and create love.
I will nurture myself.
I know that I am worthy of love and allow that worthiness to come my way.

"Never let your sense of morals prevent you from doing what is right."

~ ISAAC ASIMOV

February 16

RELATIONSHIPS

- Be **AWARE** to consider your own way of communicating with your partner.
- Pay attention to your own behavior and body language.
- Be **ALERT** and ask is there a lot of anger, frustration, and lack of communication?
- Are your mental, spiritual, physical needs met?
- How **AWARE** are the listening skills between you and your partner?

February 17

STALKERS AND ABUSIVE PARTNERS

Obsessional Stalker...

- A prior relationship exists between the victim and the stalker which includes the following:
- The stalking behavior begins after the relationship went sour.
- Can't let go. Angry.

Obsessional Intimacy Stalker...

- The delusion that the victim loves them.
- Obsessed with their love and think victim returns it.
- Pursues an intimate relationship with person they perceive as their only true love.
- Wants to rescue the person from how he/she perceives others.

February 18

- If you know who is stalking you, report to local law enforcement.
- STOP and **AVOID** all contact and communication with that person.
- Call the police and file a crime report. Keep report file number in a safe place. Be **AWARE** that this is your report case number.
- When making a supplemental report, tell the officer the report case number assigned to the original report.
- You will also need this number for the restraining or Emergency Protective Order.

February 19

- File for an Emergency Protective Order (restraining order), at your local Superior Court.
- Be **AWARE** and prepared to seek temporary safety at a shelter or with others if you are in imminent danger.
- Below list court and police phone numbers, and any emergency contacts for future use.

Today's Exercise...

I will learn to let go of past events.
I forgive myself.
I will know how to react in a healthy way.
I will stop trying to be perfect for others.
I will forgive myself.

February 20

If you feel you are being stalked (unexpectedly showing up at your job, sending unwanted messages to your phone or computer, showering you with unwanted gifts, repeatedly calling and hanging up, following your social network sites, showing up at places you hang out), record those incidents and inform law enforcement, family, friends, work colleagues.

List below any incident, time, date, location.

Maintain a journal and keep in a safe place.

February 21

HOME SECURITY

- Bodyguards and security staff ensure that their clients' homes are properly addressed with security measures. They shred vital documents and **AVOID** throwing away any identifying mail such as personal information, credit card numbers.
- They advise their clients to place alternate addresses on personal checks and business cards, such as a post office box or agent's office.
- Secret Service confirms identification of all repairmen, delivery, service, and salesmen prior to permitting entry into the White House. They ask and confirm if president made the call. Are you **AWARE** if you do the same?

February 22

George Washington (February 22, 1732 – December 14, 1799), was the first president and one of the founding fathers of the United States (1789–1797), the commander-in-chief of the Continental Army during the American Revolutionary War.

DRIVING

- If Washington had a car, he would give himself the presidential treatment to have his bodyguards circle well-lit streets a few times before going home to the White House to see if anyone was following him or lurking about the White House or garage.
- His bodyguards would be **ALERT** to check rearview mirrors often.
- He would go straight to an emergency location, or a 24-hour location, or an open and populated area, if he felt in danger.
- He would be **ALERT** that his automatic garage door immediately closed after driving in and perimeter lighting operating.

February 23

OFFICE SECURITY

- Give your office the presidential treatment.
- Central reception should handle and be properly trained for visitors and packages.
- Office staff should be **ALERT** for suspicious people, parcels, and packages that do not belong in the area.
- Establish key, lock and visitor control.
- Advise personnel, manager, and security of stalker.
- Be **AWARE** that restraining orders can be filed for work, school, or other personal locations (relatives), the stalker may be aware of or has been to.

February 24

OUT AND ABOUT

Be AWARE...

- That con artists and stalkers watch people, their habits, and vulnerabilities
- That they watch their movements, their lack of **ALERTNESS, AWARENESS,** and their vulnerable signs of being an easy victim

Today's Resolution...

WHEREAS, I am my own bodyguard! I walk with assurance and confidence.

WHEREAS, I will walk at a steady pace with shoulders back, stand erect, head high, looking around.

*WHEREAS, I am always **ALERT** and **AWARE** of my surroundings and suspicious people at all times.*

WHEREAS, I will use my five senses.

*WHEREAS, I will be **ALERT** and **AWARE** of my surroundings when I need to plan an escape route, or which streets to use whether I am on foot or driving.*

_____   _____

Signature   Date

February 25

- Have it clear (visualize), in your mind your routes of escape and **AWARENESS** plans so that high anxiety won't cloud your common sense and judgment.

- Always have a phone with you and within easy reach so you are able to use it.

- Always let someone know where you are going, the routes, and if possible, an approximate time of return.

- Carry sound alarms or whistle.

- Be **AWARE** and cautious with the use of pepper spray.

- Remember, protective weapons can be a false sense of security.

- Know and practice *The Unique Triple A*™ strategies.

- **AVOID** shortcuts, alleys, less-populated areas.

- **AVOID** stairways and dark areas around them.

- **AVOID** being caught alone in unpopulated areas.

February 26

PEPPER SPRAY

- Even bodyguards are properly trained and know when and how to use defensive weapons. Be **AWARE** of their use and proper handling.
- Be **AWARE** and **ALERT** to wind/weather factors (spray could blow back in your face), trigger-lock issues (accidental discharge), and the chance of exploding in extremely hot weather or near flames.
- There are laws and restrictions in some states.
- Most importantly, be **AWARE** to ask yourself the following questions: Is it still in your purse or pocket when you need it NOW? Where is the nozzle pointed? You or the suspect?
- Be **AWARE** to check date of purchase, shelf life, and list below.

February 27

PHONE STALKING, UNWANTED CALLS

- Are you **AWARE** that the electronic version of stalking (cyberstalking), whether online or by cell phone, often results from those who reveal too much personal information by either via e-mail or social media, such as Twitter, Facebook, chat rooms, and matchmaking sites?
- Do you have caller ID on all phones?
- Please consider a burner phone as an alternate safety phone (see GLOSSARY).

February 28

What Would The President Do?...

- Have vehicle parked and secured in well-lit and populated areas with security alarm activated.
- **AVOID** parking lots where car doors must be left unlocked and keys surrendered; otherwise surrender only the ignition key.
- Keep doors locked while driving.
- Equip the gas tank with a locking gas cap and hood-locking device controlled from inside the vehicle.
- Be **ALERT** and **AWARE** of surroundings and visually check inside, outside, and under vehicle before entering.
- Press the panic button on his presidential limousine key fob and escape to safety with his bodyguards.

February 29

- When traveling by vehicle, plan ahead.
- Be **AWARE** of 24-hour emergency locations, such as police stations, fire departments, hospitals, convenience stores.
- Be **ALERT** and use/change a different schedule and route of travel often.
- If followed, drive to a police station, fire department, or busy shopping center. Press your panic button on your remote or sound the horn to attract attention.
- Be **ALERT** for vehicles that appear to be following you. Check rearview mirror often, as well as cars around you.
- Be **AWARE** when parked in the residence's garage, turn the garage light on and lock the vehicle and garage door.
- Do you have interior garage lights that automatically turn on when garage door opens? Are they properly functioning?

BONUS SAFETY TIP

It's Not Your Fault. At an estimated rate of 1.4 million cases (including men and women) each year, stalking behavior may include phone calls, letters, gifts, snooping around your private life, tailing, threatening, or endangering, and vandalizing or stealing.

- Keep a diary or notebook handy to jot down any text messages/e-mails, voicemails, videos, letters, photos, postcards, phone calls, unwanted gifts, personal contact.
- Note witnesses, stalker's statements, date and time, location, and details of what happened.
- Remember to be **AWARE** that stalking is not your fault. It can be helpful to talk to a counselor or family to get emotional support.

"Nothing or anyone has any power over me other than that which I give it through my conscious thoughts."

~ TONY ROBBINS

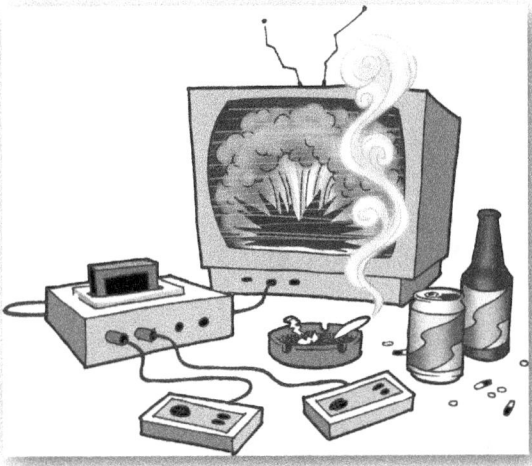

March

MARCH MADNESS

———

Youth Violence

March 1

FOR THE PARENTS

- Help yourself and family by making them safe from violence.
- Work with your own children, with other kids you care about, and with teens and adults you care about to be **ALERT, AVOID, AWARE,** and reduce the risk that you or someone you love will fall victim to violence.

NOTE:

Be **ALERT,** Daylight Saving Time starts 2:00 a.m. on the second Sunday in March. Clocks are adjusted to spring forward one hour. Don't forget to change carbon monoxide and smoke alarm batteries.

Spring is also a great time for sales on winter and spring apparel, appliances, electronics, luggage, ski/snowboard equipment, frozen food, video games, exercise machines, bicycles, jewelry. Shop thrift stores because of spring cleaning and tax write-offs, people make donations.

March 2

Start Early...

- Even very young children can learn to be **AWARE** not to kick, hit, or bite in anger or frustration, or as a solution.
- Discipline without threats.
- "Time outs," removal of privileges, restrictions, and similar penalties are successful, violence-free strategies.

March 3

Letting children discuss their thoughts about violence helps them learn how to think through these and other issues.

- **AVOID** interrupting when listening.
- Listen carefully, openly, and comment constructively.

March 4

Teach Children...

- Ways to handle conflicts and problems without using force.
- By acting as a role model for them.
- By **AVOIDING** handling disagreements with other adults, including those close to you, in violent ways.

"Experience is the worst teacher. It gives the test before presenting the lesson."

~ VERNON LAW

March 5

Teach Children...

- To be **AWARE,** discourage, and **AVOID** name-calling and teasing.
- To **AVOID** getting out of control.
- To be **AWARE** that things can move all too quickly from "just words" to fists, knives, and even firearms.
- That bullying is wrong.
- To help them learn to say "no" to bullies and to get adult help with the situation if needed.
- To remember that words can hurt as much as a fist.

March 6

Be AWARE To…

Take a hard look at what you, your family, and your friends watch and listen to for entertainment - from action movies to cop shows, from soap operas to situation comedies, from video games to music lyrics.

What Do You Watch?…

What Do Your Children Watch, What Games Are Played?…

March 7

Be AWARE Of...

- What values do movies and media entertainment teach?
- Do they make violence appear exciting, humorous, or glamorous?
- How do characters solve problems?
- Do you watch TV with your children? Talk about how violence is handled in shows and what each of you did and didn't like.
- Are the real-life consequences of violence clear?
- Set clear limits on viewing and provide active, positive alternatives for free time.
- Are alcohol and tobacco used in home?

Are You AWARE...

...of just these partial ingredients in tobacco?

benzene (petrol solvent in fuel)
formaldehyde (used to preserve dead bodies)
ammonia (toilet cleaner)
acetone (nail polish remover)
nicotine (insecticide and chemical that causes addiction)
carbon monoxide (car exhaust fumes)

March 8

<u>Be ALERT, AWARE To…</u>

- Help your children learn and practice common courtesies.
- Teach them "please," "thank you," "excuse me," and "I'm sorry." They can help ease tensions that may lead to violence.
- Listen carefully, openly, and constructively.
- Let your children discuss their thoughts about violence.
- Help them learn how to think through what they don't understand, conflicts, and other issues.

March 9

Build A Safer Neighborhood And Child...

- Research shows that there's less crime where communities are working together.
- Help your neighborhood become or stay healthy and safe.
- Get to know your neighbors.
- You can't do it alone.
- Be **ALERT.** Join, start, or reactivate a Neighborhood Watch.
- Invest in your children. Education in early childhood development yields opportunities and exponential benefits.

*"Give a man a fish and he'll eat for a day;
teach him how to fish and he'll
never go hungry."*

~ CHINESE PROVERB

March 10

- Include discussions of ways neighbors can watch out for situations that might involve children in threats or violence.
- Consider starting a formal block-parent program so that children will have reliable, recognizable places or houses to go to in the neighborhood if they feel threatened, bullied, or scared.
- Refer to RESOURCES for crime prevention and safety education programs for children between the ages of six and ten to become engaged in their communities.
- Give children a list of emergency numbers.
- Children who carry cell phones or other electronic devices should also be **AWARE** to keep the list in their devices.

March 11

- Work together to establish safe conditions in your neighborhood, such as a physical environment that doesn't invite crime or offers opportunities for violence to brew.

- Be **ALERT, AWARE,** and **AVOID** the "Broken Window Theory,"* such as overgrown lots and properties with trash, discarded furniture, tires, appliances, illegally parked or abandoned vehicles, broken windows, trash and vandalism, or graffiti. List any in your neighborhood.

*Criminological theory of the norm-setting and signaling effect of urban disorder and vandalism on additional crime and anti-social behavior. The theory states that maintaining and monitoring urban environments in a well-ordered condition may stop further vandalism and escalation into more serious crimes.

March 12

- With a group of neighbors, scan streets, yards, alleys, playgrounds, ball fields, parks, and other areas for conditions that invite gangs, transients, or other unsafe and unsavory individuals.
- Look with a child's eye; even invite some children to go with you.
- Ask children what they see that is hazardous, dangerous, and what to **AVOID.**
- Ask your local law enforcement if they'll provide pointers or other help.
- Coordinate with your local or city/county community city officials and government departments, such as public works for assistance. List numbers/contacts here.

March 13

Promote Respect And Tolerance...

- Manage Your Anger.
- **AVOID** and resolve conflicts peacefully.
- Support safety.
- Making self and family safer from violence is, for most of us, the highest priority.
- Work with your own children, with other kids you care about, and with teens and adults you care about to reduce the risk that you or someone you love will fall victim to violence.
- Help your children to both learn and practice ways to keep arguments from becoming violent.

March 14

- Talk with your kids. It can be a powerful anti-violence weapon, especially when combined with your actions as a positive role model.

- Make it clear that you do not approve of violence as a way to handle anger or solve problems. Help them learn to think about the real consequences of violent events and entertainment.

- Ask how else a conflict can be settled, what the angry person might have done instead, what you should do to **AVOID** further conflicts, and what unseen or unspoken consequences violence might have in potential conflicts.

- Ask your child if they have seen something violent, kids fighting or bullying, and if they were involved. Listen and be **AWARE** what they say and what you say. Set up a discussion scenario, such as school bullying.

March 15

Today...

- Watch TV with your children; talk about how violence is handled in shows and what each of you did and didn't like.
- Set clear limits on viewing and provide active, positive alternatives for free time.
- Turn off television, video games, and other distractions and arrange to have family time with activities and dinner. Remember conversations?
- **AVOID** conflicts. Try to compromise and resolve issues amicably.

March 16

<u>Today…</u>

- Be **ALERT** to rehearse with your children what to do in urgent situations, like finding a weapon or being approached inappropriately by a stranger, or seeing something wrong happen.

STOP!
Don't Touch.
Leave the Area.
Tell an Adult.

- Make your home a comfortable place for your children (and their friends), to gather and feel their environment is healthy and safe.
- Help them find positive, enjoyable things to do.
- Record how the rehearsal went. What did you learn? What did your children learn? What did you become **AWARE** of?

March 17

- Encourage children to stick with friends who **AVOID** and steer clear of violence and drugs.
- Emphasize the importance of being drug free.
- Research shows use of alcohol and other drugs are closely linked with violence, including the use of guns and other weapons.
- Educate your children to **AVOID** touching a weapon, and report it immediately to you.

March 18

Do You Know What To Do?...

Sometimes it's difficult for adults to know how to react when children approach them about a real or possible danger.

- You may be a neighbor, an aunt or uncle, or a grown-up who happens to be nearby.
- Suddenly a child comes to tell you something's wrong.
- How can you handle it helpfully?
- What did they do and see?
- What were they **ALERT** and **AWARE** of?

March 19

What Would You Do If...

- ...your child tells you he/she found a weapon or a possible weapon (even if it is a toy), or describes some other immediate danger?
- ...your child comes home with a weapon he/she found?
- ...your child tells you that another child found or has a gun?

March 20

BE AWARE OF YOUR LISTENING SKILLS

- Listen carefully to the child who found the weapon.
- Be **AWARE** that the child may be excited, nervous, or scared.
- Repeat what you've heard to make sure you understand clearly.
- Kneel down if necessary to communicate at the child's height, and take what they say seriously.
- Children don't casually ask for help out of the blue.
- This is a serious issue to you and the child.
- Remind them they did the right thing in telling you.

March 21

- Make sure that your children know to **AVOID** touching firearms, and what to do if they ever find a firearm or something that might be a weapon.
- Teach them to stop, don't touch, get away, and tell a trusted adult.
- Kids are curious about firearms. Education and training may be your best weapons against curiosity. Check with your local shooting range about **minimum age requirements** for firearm safety training and range shooting. Check with local police agency or organizations for any training or education programs.

March 22

- Remind children of simple self-protection rules and not to go anywhere with someone they (and you), don't know and trust.
- Set aside time and show how and when to respond to phone calls and strangers.
- Map out safe routes of a child's favorite neighborhood destinations and school.

March 23

<u>Today's Exercise</u>...

- Teach children basic strategies for personal safety to prevent violence and reduce their risk of victimization.
- List some basic exercise strategies.

March 24

The top 10 causes of violence, in order, was conducted by the National Campaign to Stop Violence in Washington D.C. and based on interviews with youth in the nation's most violent neighborhoods.

1. the media
2. substance abuse
3. gangs
4. unemployment
5. weapons
6. poverty
7. peer pressure
8. broken homes
9. poor family environment/bad neighborhoods
10. intolerance/ignorance

<u>List Below If Any Of The Above Affect You</u> ...

Source: http://www.adherents.com/misc/violence.html

March 25

SIGNS OF GANG INVOLVEMENT

The same factors that influence youth to join gangs may be early warning signs of being involved in gang activity. Identifiers or signs of youth gang-related behaviors and activities:

- Display of tattoos/gang symbols on books, clothing.
- Changing friends. Do you know them?
- Lose interest in school and family. Truant or miss classes.
- Wears clothes that display possible colors of gang affiliation, such as shirt, hat, bandana, shoes, and shoelaces.
- Be **AWARE, ALERT** how they wear clothes. Is the hat tilted to the left or right? Do they use hand/fingers as signals? Wear pants low?
- Not all youth who display these warning signs are gang members, therefore, review the facts presented and contact your local police department's gang unit.

March 26

Build AWARENESS, Partnerships And Prevention...

- Youth violence problems are too complex for law enforcement or any single agency to resolve alone.
- Keys to solutions necessitate partnerships dedicated both to stopping youth violence before it starts, and responding effectively when it does occur.
- Stop the violence before it starts.
- Respond effectively to prevent its recurrence through prevention, intervention, and enforcement.

March 27

- Educators grappling with school violence are trying to bust up cliques and limit adolescent isolation.
- Are you **AWARE** of what your child's school does?
- Are you **ALERT** to any endorsement of dress-code policies at your child's school?
- Are you **AWARE** that one in three teenagers has experienced violence in a dating relationship?

March 28

<u>Are You AWARE That?</u>...

- Youth violence consists of various harmful behaviors that can start early and then continue into young adulthood.
- You can be a victim, an offender, or a witness to the violence.
- It includes bullying, hitting, pushing, slapping.
- These can cause more emotional and psychological harm than physical harm.
- Robbery and assault (with or without weapons) can lead to serious injury or even death.
- That coordination with neighborhood and law enforcement helps stop or decrease youth violence before it starts.

March 29

- The most common age for youth to join a gang is between 13 and 15, making early prevention efforts critical.
- Be **ALERT** to the various reasons youths join gangs, such as: money (does your child possess expensive things you didn't purchase?), peer status, sense of support/belonging, perceived sense of protection, weapon access, demonstrates an outlaw mentality and dominance.
- They are more likely to abuse drugs, engage in high-risk sexual behaviors, and experience long-term health and social consequences.
- Girls join gangs in large numbers and will likely be victims of sexual abuse, abusive partner relationships, dating violence, substance abuse.

March 30

WARNING SIGNS OF
TEEN DATING VIOLENCE

Ask your daughter/son the following questions about their dating partner:

- Are they feeling any abuse that includes physical, emotional, digital, verbal, or sexual assault?
- Does their dating partner show signs of an explosive temper, frustrations, yelling, threats, or violence to solve issues?
- Does date control what you wear, or who to spend time with?
- Is there name calling, put downs, making you feel bad about yourself, embarrassing you?
- Are there frequent calling and texting to check where you are or with whom, or other jealous behavior?
- Threats to kill themselves or self-harm if you leave?
- Forcing you to do something you don't want to do, such as drinking, drugs, unwanted sex?

March 31

Teen Dating Quiz...

- **Aggression.** Acts of violence toward animals and children, parents, friends. Lack of patience.
- **Explosive temper.** Angers quickly. Unpredictable. One minute joking around, another minute screaming in your face.
- **Intimidation.** Do you feel afraid, even with a look or gesture? Smash things or destroy property? This is a way to keep you "in line" and show who is in charge of the relationship.
- **Mood Swings.** Rapid mood swings to the point they are a different person. Sometimes referred to as the "Dr. Jekyll/Mr. Hyde" phenomenon.
- **Physically Hurting.** There are no better or worse forms of abuse. If you were pushed or your arm pulled, it's still physical pain and abuse that could become a series of extreme abuse, hitting and worse.

Be **ALERT, AWARE** what you checked off!
AVOID putting yourself in dangerous situations!

BONUS SAFETY TIP

Prevention, Intervention, and Enforcement. Raise **AWARENESS** and educate students, teachers, school administrators, counselors, school resource officers, school staff, parents, and the public on effective ways to prevent or reduce youth violence.

A "Dating Contract" for teens indicates what is unacceptable behavior and the consequences for violence and abuse when dating. Please refer to http://www.domesticviolenceprevention.org for additional information on dating contracts, how to ascertain partner's values, hobbies, goals, likes/dislikes, personality, separating, breaking up. Dating teens must have a parent present to discuss the contract and co-sign.

Everyone deserves a healthy relationship and an environment safe from violence.

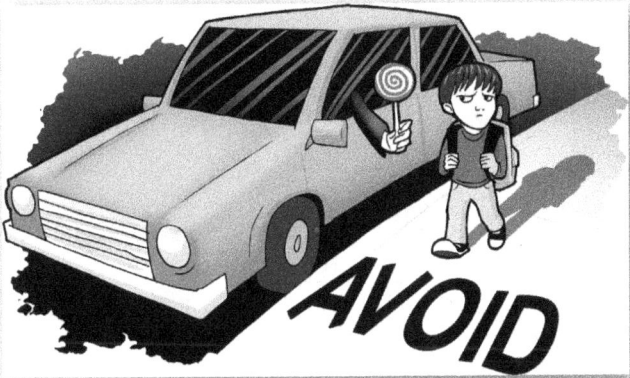

April

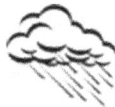

SHOWERS OF AWARENESS

———

Stranger Danger

April 1

TEACH SCHOOL SMARTS

- Make sure children take the safest routes to and from school, stores, and friends' homes. Teach child to be **ALERT** and **AWARE** to watch surroundings along the route. Teach your child to **AVOID** shortcuts to school.
- Be **AWARE** and know your child's routes to and from school, play, library, and friends' homes. Be **ALERT** that your child understands the routes, knows the street names, and can identify stores, residences. Teach them to **AVOID** walking close to curb, but in middle of sidewalk.
- If you feel your child is ready to go to school without you, walk with your child the first few days of school and pick out the safest routes.
- Does your child have ID inside clothes?
- Later, have your child walk to school with a friend or groups of other children.

April 2

- Children should check in with a parent or trusted neighbor as soon as they arrive home from school.
- **AVOID** having your child take more money than needed for school.
- Teach your child not to display money.
- Teach your child not to stay alone in a school room or in a staircase.
- **AVOID** having your child wear expensive clothing, shoes, and jewelry to school.
- Teach your child if a stranger approaches him to run away and tell a teacher.
- Ascertain school security policies and monitoring. Do security measures exist to ensure students' safety?
- Be **AWARE** if school has visitor passes that are worn by visitors and/or accompanied by a teacher or staff.

April 3

- Be **AWARE** and make sure your school has a policy that advises a parent if their child is staying late at school.
- Find out what the school's policy is for children leaving school premises with adults other than an authorized parent or guardian.
- Get together with other parents if you find these measures lacking or weak.
- Work together with school officials and law enforcement on Crime Prevention Through Environmental Design (CPTED), approaches to deter criminal activity.
- List school and police contacts below.

April 4

TEACH STREET SMARTS

Today...

- Show how to **AVOID** trouble. Teach and communicate.
- Tell them how to **AVOID** places that could be dangerous, and situations where trouble might lurk, such as vacant buildings, alleys, new construction, and wooded areas.
- Teach them to **AVOID** playing or hanging around in such public areas such as bathrooms or elevators.
- Show children safe places they can go in the neighborhood in an emergency.
- Have them be **AWARE** of a trusted neighbor's house, or emergency (fire, police, and hospital), locations.
- Teach them to always use crosswalks and obey the traffic lights when crossing the street.

April 5

- Teach children to go to a store clerk, security guard, or police officer for help if they are lost in a mall or anywhere else.
- If child or teen has a cell phone, be **ALERT** and check for any GPS programs and their usage.
- Teach them its usage.
- Teach children to walk confidently and to be **ALERT** and **AWARE** of their surroundings.
- **AVOID** shortcuts, alleys, unknown locations.
- Encourage children to **AVOID** walking and playing alone, but with friends.

NOTE:

Easter varies between March 22 and April 25, based on the lunar calendar, followed by Passover. Some religions celebrate using either the Julian or Gregorian calendars.

April 6

TEACH CHILDREN HOW TO RESPOND

Subject to age and circumstances, your children should know what to do and where to go when feeling threatened.

- Teach them police are their friends and will protect them.
- A child should also know to run and seek out a trusted teacher, neighbor, or a friend's parent. Know to report trouble right away.
- Instruct your children not to give out address or phone number to anyone, unless they are in one of the safe places, and that person is calling either police or you on their behalf.
- Teach what to do if child thinks, feels, or sees he is being followed or in danger. Yell as loud as they can for help, or go to the nearest safe place and tell a worker what happened, that they are frightened, and to call the police. Safe places include an open business, a neighbor you and your child know, fire, or police department. Are any along a school route?

April 7

- Teach them to **AVOID** being near a curb where strangers in a car can pull up next to them. Tell them to walk in center of sidewalk, but be courteous to pedestrians.
- Teach them to **AVOID** getting close to a car with a stranger.
- Teach them not to accept rides or anything from strangers.
- Teach them not to talk to strangers.
- Teach children to stay outside where help can see them, and stay where others can see them.

April 8

TEACH EMERGENCY ASSISTANCE

- Teach them how to dial "9-1-1" or other emergency numbers used in your area.
- Teach them to memorize their address, area code, and phone number.
- Let them be **AWARE** how to contact you at work.
- Let them be **AWARE** how to contact a trusted friend, relative.
- Keep a list of emergency phone numbers, and a close relative or friend's number posted near all the phones in your house.
- List numbers here as other "go to" references.

April 9

PARENTS AND HOME SMART

- Teach them to always have their key ready before they approach the door. Be **ALERT** to their surroundings.
- Teach them to always lock the door behind them.
- Once inside, instruct them not to open door to strangers and never tell anyone they are home alone.

Strangers...

- Instruct children what to do when approaching their house and a stranger is seen near the front door, driveway, etc.
- Tell them to **AVOID** the stranger, **AVOID** going into house, and **AVOID** talking or going near stranger.
- Instruct them to go to neighbor to call police.

April 10

- Be **ALERT** and **AWARE** that your child has all the safety equipment and is wearing a certified safety helmet before they ride.
- Be **ALERT** and **AWARE** to go over all laws regarding bicycle rules and responsibilities.
- Be **ALERT** and **AWARE.** Inspect brakes, tire pressure, and handlebars.
- Even during daytime, wearing something reflective can help deter accidents.
- Is bicycle correct size for your child?
- Check local fire departments. Some fire departments register bicycles.
- List bicycle information below, such as make, model, serial number.

April 11

STRANGER DANGER SMART

Today...

- Teach children that no one, not even someone they know, has the right to touch them in a way that makes them feel uncomfortable.
- Tell them they have the right to say "NO," yell as loud as possible, "STOP," "LEAVE ME ALONE," kick, bite, hit, and run away.

SAY NO!
GET AWAY!
TELL SOMEONE!

- Teach them to be **ALERT, AWARE,** and to **AVOID** dangerous situations.
- Give them a "special password" that is shared only with parents and children. Should a stranger tell them a parent asked to take them home, they must have that password.

April 12

PARENT'S RESPONSIBILITIES AT PARKS

Always be **ALERT** and **AWARE.** Keep your children in sight at all times. Adult supervision is important, but accidents do occur even when being watchful. To help prevent scraps, bruises, cuts, parents should:

- Inspect equipment for hazards and hidden sharp items, such as razor blades, nails, and bent forks before child plays on them. Inspect for bolts that stick out, loose connections, splinters.
- Be **AWARE** of spaces between bars, such as ladder steps where a child could fall through or get stuck.
- Be **ALERT** if equipment looks worn or in need of repair. **AVOID** child playing on it and attempt to contact a park or maintenance employee to let them be **AWARE** of the hazard. Be sure to list the hazardous park to **AVOID** until it is repaired.

April 13

PARENTS AND PLAYING SMART

- Teach your child to **AVOID** playing or riding bike in deserted areas, alleys, and vacant lots.
- Teach your child to be **AWARE** and lock their bikes at school or wherever else they park it.
- Teach your child about the buddy system, being with friends in play at playgrounds, parks, school.
- Teach them not to play alone.
- Teach your child to **AVOID** going to public restrooms alone or playing near them.
- Teach them what to do if a stranger approaches them.
- What playgrounds or parks does your child go to? List information below.

April 14

PUBLIC RESTROOMS SMART

Many malls and stores place restrooms at the end of long service corridors in less desirable areas or close to stockrooms.

- Be **ALERT** and **AWARE** that isolation makes these areas potential sites for anything from robbery to sexual assault.
- Pick restrooms in well-lit and well-trafficked areas.
- Always accompany children to the restroom.

April 15

GUIDE ON BABYSITTERS/PROVIDERS

- Use a friend's, neighbor's or relative's babysitter, if possible.
- If you hire someone you don't know, use extreme caution when selecting a babysitter, (including preschool or day care center).
- Ask for several references: past employers, teachers, counselors, relatives, friends, neighbors.
- Be **AWARE** to check their references and have face-to-face meetings with them before you make a decision.
- Be **ALERT** to observe their interaction with your children. Look for mature and responsible people who listen and respond well to your children, and appear relaxed and happy with them. Be specific about your expectations. Will this person become frustrated or angry if the baby cries?

April 16

- If the sitter is not an adult, you should also meet his/her parents.
- If you have made a tentative selection, you should check all references carefully. Assure those references that their comments will not be revealed to anyone, including the sitter. Ask them if they believe that the sitter possesses the demeanor, responsibility, and qualifications to care for children, and if they would hire this person to care for their children. Be **ALERT** and **AWARE** if anything said by a reference makes you feel uncomfortable.
- Ask yourself the following questions:
- Does this person know to call someone immediately if they become frustrated while caring for the baby? Have I told this person that a baby should never be shaken?
- List brief comments here.

April 17

The Arrival Of The Babysitter...

- Ask babysitter to arrive at least fifteen minutes before you leave.
- While giving babysitter instructions, note demeanor and listening skills.
- Ensure babysitter is **AWARE** of locations for telephones, first-aid kits, emergency numbers, your contact numbers, medical needs (asthma), all exits in case of an emergency. If you have a second-story, have an emergency ladder available.
- Ensure that the sitter fully understands specific responsibilities that include:
  - Never leave children alone at any time.
  - Be **AWARE, ALERT**, watchful.
  - Daily routines (homework, eating, TV).
  - Food allergies, medication dosage.
  - Never advise callers he/she is the babysitter. Take a message.

April 18

<u>Responsibility Advice To Babysitter</u>...

- Never open the door for anyone. All doors/windows remain secured and locked.
- Remember, the babysitter is responsible for your children. Having other children in your home who play or visit your children need supervision as well. Talk with babysitter about this. Authorize who may visit.
- Children should be watched closely while awake, especially if taken outside.
- Children should be checked regularly after they have gone to sleep.
- Let babysitter be **AWARE** of rules associated with use of your belongings (telephones, computers, appliances).
- Babysitter's friends are not authorized to visit your home.
- Parents are responsible to ensure that children understand that the babysitter is in charge and that they are expected to follow all family rules.

April 19

Returning Home To Babysitter...

- Even if you are tired, be **ALERT** and check on your children.
- Discuss children's behavior and activity.
- Was anything out of the ordinary or concerning to the babysitter?
- Ascertain phone calls and messages.
- Ascertain solicitors (never answer door).
- Ascertain visitors, child's friends (unless authorized by you, they are not invited into home).
- List brief comments here.

NOTE:

In the state of New York, Kieran's Law allows parents to request fingerprint background checks of in-house caregivers who provide care for more than 15 hours per week. Check to see if your state has a similar law.

April 20

<u>After The Babysitter Has Left</u>...

- Be **AWARE** and **ALERT** to discuss with your children how they felt with the babysitter, what activities they did.
- Ask if anything made them feel afraid or uncomfortable.
- Ask if visitors did in fact come into the house.
- Ask if they would like the babysitter to return again.
- List brief comments here.

April 21

FIREARM OWNER
SAFETY RESPONSIBILITIES

- Store weapons appropriately and safely (in gun safety cabinets).
- Keep them unloaded and locked up. Hide the keys. Lock weapons and ammunition in separate locations. If ammunition is easy to get to, children will learn very fast how to load an unloaded gun.
- Ask neighbors, or homes child frequents, to do the same if they own guns.
- Talk to your children about guns, gun safety, and what they should, or should not do, around guns.
- Teach young children not to touch guns, and to tell an adult if they find one.

STOP!
DON'T TOUCH.
LEAVE THE AREA.
TELL AN ADULT.

April 22

SETTING RULES/PREPARING HOME ALONE

For various reasons there are times when parents can't always be there when children come home from school, but are they ready to be "Home Alone," and at what age? Here are some suggested brief basic maturity tests.

Give opportunities. Help them to practice independent problem-solving skills. Help build child's confidence to complete these tasks. By age three, your child should be able to dress himself with help for buttons/zippers, but motor skills will improve in time. Toddlers can put their clean clothes into drawers, dirty ones into a hamper. Resist the urge to clean up after child. Two-year-olds can put away their own toys. Preschoolers can match socks, and 6 to 8-year-olds can fold laundry. By late elementary school, kids should be capable of washing their own clothes.

April 23

Today...

Give chores. Your child lives in your home, so have child take some responsibility for keeping it clean. A toddler can help make beds, and in elementary school, add sweeping, vacuuming, and mopping as chores.

At first, leave your child alone for short periods and see how child handles being on own. Talk about concerns and any fears child has. Agree on ground rules for cooking, having friends over, and set time for homework. Assign tasks to accomplish to keep child busy.

Observation Notes...

April 24

FOR THE CHILDREN

BE BIKE SMART

- Be **ALERT, AWARE,** and obey all traffic signs.
- Always wear your safety helmet.
- Look both ways before you pull out into the street.
- Be **AWARE** and use hand signals when stopping or making a turn.
- Be courteous to pedestrians. When walking bike across street, let pedestrians go first.
- Even during the day, always wear something reflective.
- Check with parent for state laws that require front and rear lights.
- Be **AWARE** and use a two-lock locking system to secure bike. Two locks increase time, tools, for thief to defeat. Primary lock should be a U-shaped with flat key, and secondary lock, a self-locking cable.

April 25

STRANGER DANGER SMART

- Be **AWARE** of dangerous situations. If a stranger asks you for help or to keep a "special secret," it could be a dangerous situation.
- Be **ALERT, AWARE, AVOID,** and never accept rides, candy, gifts, money, or medicine from a stranger.
- If they tell you that your mom or dad sent them or they are injured, sick, need finding a pet, or threaten you - run away.
- **AVOID** the stranger by stepping back, scream, run away, and tell someone.
- If something does happen, yell as loud as possible, "STOP," "LEAVE ME ALONE," kick, bite, hit, and run away.

SAY NO!
GET AWAY!
TELL SOMEONE!

April 26

- Be **ALERT, AWARE, AVOID,** and never get close to a car if a stranger calls out to you for directions or anything else. It is easy for a stranger to pull you into a car.
- Be **ALERT, AWARE, AVOID,** and never go anywhere with someone.
- They must have your parent's permission and the Secret Password you and your parents shared with you.
- If a stranger in a car bothers you, turn and run in the opposite direction.
- It is not easy for a car to change directions suddenly.
- Be **ALERT** if the car continues to follow you.
- Yell out for help.
- If a stranger tries to follow you on foot or tries to grab you, run away, scream, and make lots of noise.
- Carry a whistle or alarm to make noise.

April 27

AT HOME SMART

- Call parent as soon as you get home from school.
- Never open your house door to anyone you do not know. Tell them parents cannot come to the door and **AVOID** engaging in conversation.
- If you are home alone keep the radio or television on. Never tell anyone you are home alone.
- Be **ALERT** and **AWARE** to always keep doors and windows locked when home alone.
- Never give your name or address to a stranger, or volunteer family vacation plans or other information about your home.
- Learn how to dial 9-1-1 with a parent and when to use it.
- Call the police (9-1-1), if a stranger tries to talk you into opening the door or tries to get in.
- Keep a list of phone numbers that parents gave you, such as work numbers, relative, neighbor, emergency, etc.

April 28

- **AVOID** telling strangers or anyone on the phone you don't know that you are home alone.
- Tell them parents cannot come to the phone and **AVOID** engaging in conversation.
- Ask for a call back phone number.
- **AVOID** telling someone you do not know your phone number, name, or address. HANG UP.
- Have parents help you be **AWARE** of Caller ID.
- If someone scares you on the phone and your parents are not home, hang up. Use Caller ID to screen calls.
- If someone calls you and says bad things over the phone, hang up. **AVOID** and do not talk to them.

April 29

AT PLAY AND OUT AND ABOUT

- **AVOID** going to public rest rooms by yourself. Go with a parent or trusted adult.
- Be **ALERT, AWARE, AVOID** strangers who are hanging around restrooms or the playground, and strangers who want to play with you and your friends. Run to the nearest person you can find (police officer, adult, opened store).
- **AVOID** showing money in public. Carry only what is necessary and keep it in a pocket until needed.
- **AVOID** hitchhiking. NEVER HITCHHIKE.
- **AVOID** playing or hanging around in such public areas as bathrooms or elevators. **AVOID** stairways, out-of-the-way corridors, dimly-lit areas, dense shrubbery that hide people.
- **AVOID** and NEVER touch a firearm.

STOP!
LEAVE THE AREA.
TELL AN ADULT.

April 30

SCHOOL BUS SMART

Waiting...

- Wait with friends. Stay away from the curb.
- Whether sitting on bench or standing, be **AWARE, ALERT** around and behind you. Pay attention to approaching bus and let it come to a complete stop before boarding. **AVOID** displaying money. **AVOID** pushing or crowding those getting on or off the bus.

On the Bus...

- Face forward when sitting and near driver.

Exiting the Bus...

- Take five giant steps away out of danger zone.

April 31

Aa   We will be **AWARE, ALERT** and **AVOID.**

Bb   We will stand up to **Bullying** and safe schools.

Cc   We will practice **Crime** Prevention.

Dd   We will prepare **Disaster** kits for home, car.

Ee   We will implement an **Emergency** plan.

Ff   We will visit a **Fire** station and learn fire safety.

Gg   We will lock and secure all **Guns.**

Hh   We will plan **Home** emergency & safety scenario(s).

Ii   We will be **ALERT** to the dangers on the **Internet.**

Jj   We will celebrate **July** 4th safely and obey all laws.

Kk   We will teach our **Kids** safety and prevention skills.

Ll   We will always **Lock** up and put away bikes and tools.

Mm   We will **AVOID** playing with **Matches.**

Nn   We will join or start a **Neighborhood** Watch.

Oo   We will practice **Our** *The Unique Triple A*™ strategies.

Pp   We will be responsible and take care of our **Pets.**

Qq   We will create **Quality** of life programs.

Rr   We will always wear a helmet when **Riding** bikes.

Ss   When in **Sun**, we will wear sunscreen.

Tt   We will **AVOID** alcohol, drugs, and **Tobacco** products.

Uu   We will dispose **Unused**/expired prescription drugs.

Vv   We will always buckle up when in a **Vehicle.**

Ww   We will always be watchful with our kids near **Water.**

Xx   We will pay **Xtra** attention when we are out and about.

Yy   We will install and maintain smoke alarms twice a **Yea**r.

Zz   Use **Zip**-Ties on luggage for additional security.

BONUS SAFETY TIP

Establish a system and make time to discuss "safety tool-box talks." Select any of the topics in the month of April and arrange a family meeting to discuss and emphasize its **AWARENESS** and how it offers children strategies to **AVOID** dangerous situations. Make it entertaining, but educational.

If you choose to discuss the "Home Alone," subject, remember age isn't the only factor to consider in leaving a child home alone. Consider how your child handles various situations and ask the following:

How does your child handle unexpected situations? How calm does your child stay when things don't go as planned?

Does your child understand and follow rules?

Can your child understand and follow safety measures? Does your child show signs of responsibility with things like homework, household chores, and following directions?

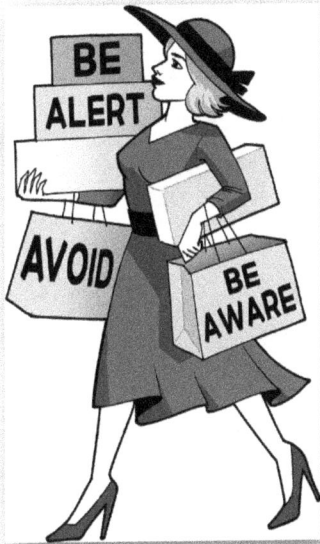

May

MOM'S DAY

—

Out & About

May 1

SITUATIONAL AWARENESS

- Is when you see something that just doesn't look right and it puts you on **ALERT** to react and/or assess a potential threat.
- Be **AWARE, ALERT** to **AVOID,** and eliminate potential dangers. Develop proper psychological habits.
- Think and practice safety.

Today's Exercise...

- Think about the five most dangerous situations that could occur in your life. Only you know what circumstances are potential dangers for you.
- Take into account your neighborhood, work, travel, car. Visualize yourself in these situations, then figure out ways how to protect yourself. Use *The Unique Triple A*™ strategies.
- List them on a piece of paper or journal.

May 2

Summarize what you wrote yesterday. Congratulations on your continuing committed safety resolutions.

1. _____

   _____

   _____

2. _____

   _____

   _____

3. _____

   _____

   _____

4. _____

   _____

   _____

5. _____

   _____

   _____

May 3

OUT & ABOUT AND SHOPPING

- Be **ALERT** and **AWARE** to your surroundings, and anything or anyone suspicious.
- Make yourself a "tough" target.
- Walk purposely with confidence, head held high. Look around with confidence.
- Walk with shoulders straight, not bent.
- Use your head and be proactive in common sense approaches to personal safety.
- Give appearance you are totally **AWARE** of your surroundings and know who is nearby.
- Look people in the eyes instead of turning away or head bent down.
- Recognize, eliminate, and **AVOID** potential and dangerous situations.
- Do the buddy system and shop with friends.

We always hold hands.
If I let go, she shops."

~ HENRY YOUNGMAN

May 4

- **AVOID** behaviors that can put you at risk of being victimized.
- **AVOID** getting into a verbal exchange that can escalate into a conflict or physical altercation (someone takes your parking space or bumps into you), injuries, or worse.
- **AVOID** using a purse, especially with straps, if possible.
- Try a zippered "fanny pack." You don't need a big purse to carry the "sink."
- If you must carry a shoulder bag, shorter straps allow you to keep your purse close to you. Keep your arm over it to keep it snug to your body.
- If snatched, **AVOID** fighting for your purse.
- Be **ALERT** and try to use the buddy system by shopping with friends.

May 5

- **AVOID** wearing/displaying expensive jewelry.
- You may want attention, but might get the wrong attention.
- If you still want to wear your diamond ring, turn it around to face palm.
- **AVOID** carrying more than you need or can handle.
- Carry only amount of packages that do not obstruct your view or hinder your movements
- Carrying more packages decreases your view to be **ALERT,** and **AWARENESS** of your surroundings. Makes you an easier target and decreases **AWARENESS** to **AVOID** potential dangerous persons and situations.
- Carrying more packages decreases **AWARENESS** to look for your parked car, increases and creates opportunities for surprise attacks, robberies.

May 6

- Carry a minimum amount of cash, checks, and credit cards as needed for that day.
- Carry keys and ID separately from purse.
- In the event of a theft, the thief won't have your home address and a set of house keys.
- **AVOID** carrying your Social Security card or PIN numbers.
- Find out if the stores and malls you use to shop have escorts or security escorts to help you to your vehicle.
- **AVOID** restrooms at end of long corridors in less desirable areas or close to stockrooms. Isolation creates potential dangerous situations.

May 7

- **AVOID** carrying a load of packages that hinder your **ALERTNESS** and **AWARENESS.**
- **AVOID** shopping 'til you drop.
- Fatigue decreases your **ALERTNESS** and **AWARENESS,** and you will not be able to **AVOID** potential dangerous situations or keep careful track of your shopping bags or other packages.
- Fatigue decreases your ability to be **ALERT** and **AWARE** to check your receipts.
- When entering a mall, be **ALERT** and **AWARE** to use store directory. This decreases shopping time looking for a store and decreases an opportunity for a criminal to look for lost, inattentive, or confused patrons that are easy targets.

May 8

At the Register Counter...

- Check receipts to see whether your full credit card number appears. If a receipt has your full number on it, take a pen and thoroughly scratch it out. Immediately contact and advise store manager and ascertain if this is their store policy and advise of potential identity theft.
- Be **ALERT** and **AWARE** of your credit card at the register. **AVOID** letting it out of your sight.
- Be sure it is immediately returned to you, and double check that you have your credit cards and checkbook after you paid for your items.
- Be **ALERT** that your purse/wallet is secured before leaving counter.
- **AVOID** being distracted by your cell phone, chatting or anything else during register transactions and while shopping.

May 9

PARKING

- Keep your car in good running condition. Make sure there's enough gas to get where you're going and back (never let gas tank get less than one-quarter full).
- Be **ALERT** and leave home early to shop.
- Park car near stores, entryways, or where you can be seen from the street.
- If you shop until late hours, at least you will have your car nearby and in lit areas.
- **AVOID** waiting until closing time to leave.
- Consider leaving before dark to increase your **AWARENESS** of the parking lot surroundings for potential dangerous persons or situations.
- Keep belongings out of sight when you park your car. Eliminate temptation for criminal opportunists.

May 10

- When parking, **AVOID** stairwells, out-of-the way corridors, elevators, poorly lighted areas, and corners that easily conceal a person.

- When parking, always be **ALERT** and **AWARE** where the closest exits are located in case of fire, emergency, and your escape from danger. **AVOID** parking next to vans.

- Be **AWARE** and **ALERT** when using underground parking garages. Park close to entries and **AVOID** parking in isolated areas.

- Be **AWARE** that your doors are locked and windows rolled up tightly, even if you are gone a short time.

- **AVOID** being distracted and be **ALERT** and **AWARE** of surroundings while exiting, entering, and securing your car.

May 11

- **AVOID** leaving any valuables in plain view. Lock them in the trunk. Do so before leaving home or reaching your final destination to **AVOID** observation of any would-be thieves or opportunists who might take notice.
- Consider using an anti-theft device such as a steering wheel lock.
- **AVOID** storing a key under fender, tire.
- If you have to run errands or shop at night, park in well-lighted and well-traveled areas.
- Identify and ascertain malls or stores that use escort services. If shopping alone, ask for an escort to your car, should you want one.
- Some shopping malls provide valet parking. **AVOID** leaving values in car and handing over all keys to valet.
- Look for malls that have security patrol.

May 12

Parking Attendants and Valet Services...

- **AVOID** leaving important papers, briefcases in plain view, in glove compartment and trunk.
- **AVOID** giving all your keys, including house key, to parking attendants. Keys can be duplicated.
- If you have separate car keys for trunk, glove compartment, and ignition, give ignition key only to attendant.
- Does your ignition key open both glove compartment and trunk?
- Use an alternate address or post office box address on car documents, such as registration, insurance. **AVOID** marking or leaving an ID tag on your key chain with your name, address for opportunists.

May 13

Returning to Car...

- Overexposed? Not you. Too many packages being carried hinder your **AWARENESS** and expose you to danger.
- Exposing packages or gifts on the back seat or covering them will not fool a thief, only yourself.
- Be **ALERT, AWARE** of opportunities for car prowlers and package thefts when your packages and gifts are overexposed in view.
- If you will be traveling from one shopping location to another, keep your gifts in your trunk, locked and secured. **AVOID** carrying all your packages from several shopping trips that will hinder your vision and attendance to **AWARENESS.**
- Have your keys ready in hand with keys protruding in-between fingers for defense.
- Always be **ALERT** and **AWARE** of your surroundings before approaching your car.

May 14

- Be **AWARE** that carrying too many packages not only hinders your **ALERTNESS** to your surroundings, but you will have to set them down to get your keys out of your purse. During those moments of distraction, you become a potential victim. Less packages, keys in hand **AVOIDS** potential danger.

- **AVOID** walking close to other parked vehicles and vans.

- Be **AWARE** to walk in the center of the access way against the direction of traffic.

- If you see someone loitering near your car, **AVOID** (be **ALERT** to use the panic button on your remote key), and return to store for help.

- If you use a keyless entry remote, **AVOID** unlocking car until you see your vehicle.

- Check inside, outside, under, and around your car before entering.

- Lock the doors IMMEDIATELY upon entering your car.

- Leave immediately. You can always place packages in trunk at a safer area.

May 15

When returning to your car, remember *The Unique Triple A*™ strategies:

ALERT. Recognize potential dangerous situations.
AWARE. Of your surroundings.
AVOID. Being vulnerable and in danger.

In summary, remember **E.L.F.S.**

Enter the car.
Lock the doors.
Fasten seat belts.
Scram.

NOTE:

In the United States, **Armed Forces Day** is celebrated on the third Saturday in May. It falls near the end of Armed Forces Week, which begins on the second Saturday of May and ends on the third Sunday of May. President Harry S. Truman led the effort to establish a single holiday for citizens to come together and thank all military (Army, Navy, Marine Corps, Air Force) members for their patriotic service in support of our country.

May 16

BE ALERT

- Three bad habits victims have are denial, complacency, and apathy.

- "It will never happen to me." Be **ALERT** to consider, "It can and may happen to me." Be **ALERT** to be mentally prepared.

- Look at your safety resolution lists. How might you have eliminated those situations?

- It is amazing how many dangerous situations you will be able to completely eliminate by thinking/planning ahead.

- Be **ALERT** to your gut or sixth sense that something is wrong.

- It's great you carry pepper spray, a cell phone, or a whistle, but if you are attacked or feel something is wrong, can you access them quickly? Do you know how to safely use pepper spray?

- Do you know where you are, the names of the streets you are on, when you call for help?

May 17

BE AWARE

- Always be **AWARE** of your surroundings and persons around you.
- Be **AWARE** if your space (COLOR CODE ZONES) being invaded by a stranger. Walk with purpose. Be **AWARE** of your body language.
- Be **AWARE** of body language of suspicious person.
- Be **AWARE** of assuming the leave-me-alone stance and positioning to strangers.
- Angle your body to about 45-degrees which makes you a smaller target. You can easily rotate hips into a kick or hand strike, if necessary.
- Feet are shoulder-width apart for balance and knees slightly bent to step quickly away or a direction without giving away your intent.
- Be **AWARE** of the best avenues of escape.

May 18

AVOID

- The "he came out of nowhere" response.
- The "he surprised me" response.
- The attacker, of course, didn't. The fact remains, they did come from somewhere.
- The attacker was there, but perhaps the victim was not **ALERT** and **AWARE** until it was too late to **AVOID**.
- **AVOID** hiding places, dense foliage, shrubbery, trees, and darkened doorways, or anyplace someone can be hidden from view.
- To really **AVOID** and secure yourself on city streets or anywhere else is to be mindful of your environment and the most vital thing you can do.

May 19

- **AVOID** flashing money on a city street, at an ATM machine, registers, and crowded areas.
- **AVOID** crowded areas (even store sales draw crowds). A pickpocket is able to take wallet, cash, or credit cards out of unsecured purses or pockets easily.
- **AVOID** being distracted.
- Be **ALERT** and **AWARE** that your purse, shopping packages, umbrella, cane, and keys are weapons to use and strike against an assailant.
- Be **AWARE** and mindful of any cues from environment that make you feel uncomfortable
- As a last resort, if you are being followed, or you feel you are likely to be attacked, toss your valuables into a government mailbox stand if one is available.

May 20

PURSES

- Let the attacker have it, as long as you get away. If an attacker attempts to grab your purse, **AVOID** fighting or holding onto it, rather than run the risk of being injured.
- If possible, wear a fanny pack.
- Grasp purses like a football player. Hug it to your ribs/chest tightly.
- Clutch bags with snap closures (held close to body), can be turned upset down to allow contents to fall out and distract attacker long enough for you to scream and escape to safety.
- Carry purse away from a street curb to **AVOID** the risk of a car or motorcycle "drive-by."
- If you must carry a purse with shoulder straps, shorten the straps so you can keep under elbow and straps don't dangle below waist. Metal chain straps cannot be cut.
- Use exposed pockets for non-valuable items. Store wallet and phone on inside secured pockets.

May 21

- That is why one should **AVOID** carrying the "kitchen sink" of family photos, more money, credit cards than needed, makeup, valuables. It's a natural instinct, these are more important to hold onto or fight for than the life that carried it all, including that expensive "name" bag.
- Keep keys in a pocket, separate from purse.
- Option: Place a dummy wallet with fake credit cards and a wad of paper in your purse. Place the real things in a wallet belt or stash in clothing.
- Perhaps you won't be as tempted to fight for the "kitchen sink."
- If you carry personal security alarms or pepper spray, place it separately from purse.
- However, be **ALERT** and **AWARE** of their usage, how and when to use (see WEAPONS).

May 22

VEHICLE

- If your vehicle breaks down, call for help on the cell phone, lock all windows and doors, and don't open the vehicle or window for anyone until help arrives.

- If your auto insurance includes tow service, call them. Some purchased or leased vehicles offer tow service as well. Check your auto insurance on tow service free mileage limitations and expiration date.

- Keep your car in good running condition, including tires (and spare), oil, water, battery, and be **ALERT, AWARE** there's enough gas to get where you're going and back (never let gas tank get less than one-quarter full).

- Be **ALERT, AWARE** to always keep your purse under the passenger seat or on the floorboard out of public view, or in trunk.

- Keep packages, purses, and valuable items in the trunk of your car, or out of view.

May 23

- Be **ALERT** to motorbike riders or drivers who target vehicles stopped in traffic, smash the passenger window, or unlocked passenger door, gain entry and grab purse that lays ATOP THE PASSENGER SEAT IN PLAIN VIEW (**AVOID** THIS). When stopped in traffic, leave enough distance between your vehicle and the vehicle in front of you. The space allows you to pull away quickly, if necessary, and if bumped from behind, it might **AVOID** your vehicle striking the one in front of you.

- Be **ALERT** your cellular telephone is near you.

- Be **ALERT** and **AWARE** of staged vehicle scams, such as the "sideswipe" and the "swoop and squat," as described in the month of July.

- When returning home at night, call ahead and have a family member watch for you.

- On the way home, check your rearview mirror often. If you feel you are being followed, **AVOID** going home and drive toward help.

May 24

Vehicle Security...

- Be **ALERT** to anti-theft devices.
- Alarm systems, kill switches, steering wheel locks can help decrease the risk of vehicle theft and opportunities for criminals.
- **AVOID** leaving anything in your vehicle. Clean out your car. A clean car can mean nothing of value inside. This includes briefcases, change, clothes, laptop computers or other electronic devices, garage door openers, purses/wallets.
- **AVOID** opportunity and temptation to criminals. Take removable stereos out of car with you.
- Be **AWARE** of anti-theft decals you can place on a window.

May 25

- Use an engraver to etch your driver's license number on different parts of your vehicle to prevent theft.
- Vehicle codes require that vehicle registration be present in car while being operated, but it should be hidden well, or you can take it with you when you exit car.
- Be **AWARE** you can use a P.O. Box or alternate address other than your home address on your vehicle registration or other paperwork.
- Make copies of registration and keep originals at home.

May 26

At Gas Stations...

- Always lock your vehicle doors and roll up windows whether you are pumping gas, paying at the pump, or paying inside the station.
- Be **ALERT** to always take keys, purse, wallet, and lock the doors while you are pumping gas.
- **AVOID** leaving valuables, purses, wallets in plain view even when you lock vehicle.
- Keep valuables out of plain view in your vehicle and lock the doors even if you are going inside for a moment. Take purse or wallet with you.

May 27

- Be **AWARE** of "sliding." Thieves drive up to the victim's car, "slide" under the view of the car owner pumping gas on the opposite side or inside paying for gas, open unlocked door, grab any valuables within reach, and drive off quickly.

- So called because of the way the criminal "slides" in below the eye level of the door and victim.

- Pick stations that are well-lit and have video surveillance cameras at the pump.

- Attempt to use gas pump nearest the attendant of the gas station.

- Be **ALERT** and **AWARE** of the surroundings and your car while you are pumping gas.

- **AVOID** letting your cell phone or other electronic devices distract you.

May 28

Memorial Day is on the last Monday of the month, so make the weekend a safe one.

Fire & Grill Safety. Clean grill of grease/dust. Check tubes leading into burner for blockages, insects, grease. Replace connectors when needed. Have correct fire extinguisher nearby.

Food Safety. AVOID food poisoning. Cook fresh poultry to 165°F, hamburgers 160°F, beef 145°F, or temperatures on packges. Refrigerate perishables within 2 hours.

Sun Safety. Wear sunscreen of at least SPF 15 or more and apply generously throughout day. Wear sunglasses, hat, and drink plenty of water.

Water Safety. AVOID alcohol when swimming or boating. Wear lifejacket on boat. Supervise children. Learn CPR. Don't swim alone.

May 29

Self-defense is not about having a degree belt and thinking you are invincible. It is about skills, common sense, and knowing when to stop an assault to get away. It is about being **AWARE** and **ALERT** to **AVOID** incidents.

One of the main focuses of martial arts training is learning and attacking an offender's sensitive vital areas of the body, such as ears, eyes, groin, nose, solar plexus, and throat. You learn how to prepare to defend and be aggressive enough to focus on these striking points, and strike hard, such as using a finger to the eye, a knee to the groin, an elbow to the nose, a fist strike to the bridge, side of, and under the nose, or a foot strike on the instep or ankle.

Yet, many women who are attacked are often not prepared to defend themselves mentally or physically, let alone conduct a foot strike, force a finger in the assailant's eye or grab the groin area to pull down quick, hard, and squeeze. Often they rely on improvised weapons, such as mace, which can be a false sense of security when you are not prepared mentally.

May 30

IMPROVISED WEAPONS

- Anything can be used when available. The key to *The Unique Triple A*™ is PAY ATTENTION to your surroundings first. These weapons are used to DISTRACT, then RUN AWAY TO SAFETY.
- Cup of hot coffee or drink to the eyes.
- An umbrella thrust to the groin, solar plexus, throat, or ribs. Maintain a distance, yet attack.
- High heels, used like a hammer or spike.
- Keys are used to stab and target sensitive, bony or fleshy areas, such as ears, face, under the chin, eyes, trachea, carotid artery, nose, solar plexus, groin, hand, and so on. Be **ALERT** that keys are readily available and should be placed in-between fingers ready as an offensive weapon.
- Pencil or ink pen thrust to the eye, hand, or throat.
- Portfolio briefcase, purse to slap across face.

May 31

A Test Of True Or False Sense Of Security…

1. Pepper sprays, stun guns, and Tasers can get stuck in the bottom of your purse?
2. Pepper sprays have an expiration date?
3. Can pepper spray aerosol canisters accidently discharge?
4. A stun gun uses high voltage, is a direct-contact weapon, used at a risk of close range. Is there a certain amount of time for an effective charge?
5. Taser guns shoot out two Taser probes about fifteen feet apart to produce a sharp electrical shock to an individual?
6. Caught off guard, an attacker can easily take these weapons and use against you?
7. They are used to DISTRACT attacker so you can run and escape?

BONUS SAFETY TIP

Women need to pay attention not only to their surroundings, but trust their instincts. Using common sense to be **ALERT, AWARE,** and **AVOID** doesn't take physical strength, size, and gender into consideration, just mental fitness. Your ultimate goal is to DISTRACT and get away, but you don't achieve that by being a meek and mild Clark Kent. You get away by pulling in a mindset of hardwired, survival instincts to attack like an enraged lioness protecting her cubs.

Being observant, and **AWARE** of a situation that might pose a threat, obeying your instincts, and empowering yourself to be a "rather safe than sorry" strategy can help to **AVOID** a potential dangerous situation.

NOTE:

Answers to May 31: 1-7, all True.

May is also Older Americans Month as designated by President Kennedy in 1963, to recognize the value of older adults and their contributions. Refer to NOVEMBER for senior citizen safety tips.

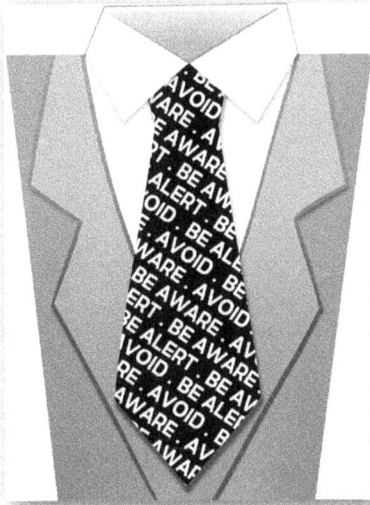

June

DAD'S DAY

———

Tie-ing One On

June 1

THINK OUTSIDE THE TIE BOX

- Remember not every situation is what it appears to be.
- An observant person can pick up on subtle cues that something is amiss.
- If a person is not **AWARE** and **ALERT**, missing those crucial instants in which a ruse may be seen for what it is, then a person becomes a victim of a crime that could have been **AVOIDABLE**.
- Instead of passing the problem to someone else, we all need to take responsibility to be **AWARE.** This starts with prevention, and ends with **AVOIDANCE**.

June 2

OUT AND ABOUT

- A wallet carried in your back pocket is an easy target for a pickpocket and can be removed without your knowledge.
- A comb in the fold of the wallet can also make you **AWARE** when someone attempts to lift your wallet. The teeth of the comb can snag inside the pocket enough to prevent the theft.

June 3

- Consider carrying your wallet in a front pocket of your pants instead of the back pocket using these preventative methods.
- **AVOID** carrying a large amount of cash and credit cards.
- Take only what you need for the day.
- Divide your cash between pockets and wallet.

June 4

For some men, the fear of appearing weak can make them forget their personal safety in a potentially dangerous situation. Remember, even the most macho martial arts person is **ALERT, AWARE,** and **AVOIDS** confrontations when they can.

- **AVOID** putting yourself at risk.
- Your primary aim should be to get away fast.
- There is no shame in doing this: it's the SMART thing to do.
- Physical self-defense should only be a last resort.
- It limits your options and commits you to a fight you could lose.
- It is not weak to walk away from violence.

June 5

ATHLETIC FACILITIES

- Use the buddy system and work out with a friend.
- **AVOID** using facilities alone, especially after dark or during off-hours.
- Become familiar with the location of facility phones.
- **AVOID** showering alone in the locker room.
- Report any suspicious incidents or persons.
- **AVOID** wearing jewelry, and secure items in locker.

June 6

ATM TRANSACTIONS

Before...

- Be **AWARE** of your total environment when driving into the parking lot.
- **AVOID** ATMs at corner of the building, rear area, blind spots, and out of public view.
- **AVOID** objects that block the line of sight, objects that can conceal persons, such as shrubbery, signs, barriers, partitions, dividers, and landscaping.
- Identify an ATM location with surveillance cameras and visibility from the surrounding area, and well-lit at night.
- Whenever possible, select an ATM that is monitored or patrolled by security.
- Maintain a small supply of deposit envelopes at home, in your car, or office. Prepare all transaction paperwork prior to your arrival at the ATM site.

June 7

During Transactions...

- **AVOID** wearing expensive jewelry, watches, or taking other valuables to the ATM.
- If you get cash – **AVOID** lingering and/or counting the money at the ATM. Put it away immediately.
- If you use a drive-up ATM, be **ALERT** and **AWARE** that your vehicle doors and windows are locked.
- While retrieving money, be **ALERT** and **AWARE**. Every few seconds look around to check out surroundings. If a situation feels uncomfortable, remove yourself from the machine and leave immediately.

After the Transactions...

- Walk immediately to car, lock it, and leave.
- When leaving, be **ALERT** and **AWARE** of the area, and that you are not being followed.

June 8

ATM CYBERCRIME

Cyber threats have become one of the most serious economic and national security challenges. Most notably were the thefts of personal data from Target, Chase, supermarket chains, and the alterations on ATMs to allow huge withdrawals, often around holidays and weekends, when extra dollars are loaded into ATMs. Though financial institutions have monitored incoming traffic, upgraded security systems for phishing and malware software attacks, and activated incident response plans, such as terminating compromised debit cards and warning their customers, be **ALERT** to your safety and criminal actions with banking activities.

The American Bankers Association recommend that consumers **AVOID** using debit or ATM cards and use credit cards (process of any fraud are not directly drawn from bank accounts); change PINS often and place a cap on ATM withdrawals. Be **ALERT** some prepaid cards do not come with deposit insurance.

Source: http://www.securityweek.com and
http://www.dhs.gov/national-cyber-security-awareness-month

June 9

BICYCLES, MOTORCYCLES

- Be **ALERT** to motorbike riders or drivers who target motorbikes stopped in traffic and attempt to remove loose or unsecured property.
- **AVOID** leaving a helmet or riding equipment on your bike after parking it.
- Park in a well-lit location, or near security camera.
- Chain and lock to a secure unmovable item when leaving it unattended.
- Besides alarms, cables, and chains, be **AWARE** of new anti-theft products, such as the disc lock mounted onto a brake disc. A locking pin goes through either a cutaway space inside disc, or one of its holes, to prevent the wheel from turning around. When selecting a locking device, be **AWARE** that some come in bright colors to help serve as a visual deterrent.

June 10

- Some alarms incorporate a current drain sensor that monitors the electrical system to detect when someone is trying to hot wire a motorcycle.

- Be **AWARE** that more expensive systems send a text message to your phone if tampered with, even if you're unable to hear the alarm.

- New designs and products, such as power supplies for cell phones and GPS devices can make every ride safer.

- Motorcycle covers can disguise and make motorcycle less likely to be targeted. Purchase one you can place a lock on to prevent removal.

- Check with your motorcycle insurance company if they offer a discount for anti-theft devices installed on your motorcycle and car.

- Be **AWARE** you have the right insurance protection for your motorcycle, if stolen.

June 11

WHAT'S IN YOUR WALLET?

- **AVOID** carrying large amounts of cash.
- Place a comb upside down inside the fold of your wallet that allows the ends to stick out (but room to fit in pocket). If a pickpocket attempt occurs, the teeth of the comb will snag inside the pocket for difficult extraction. **AVOID** wrapping rubber bands around wallet as it compresses the wallet for easy extraction.
- **AVOID** walking through large crowds or other crowded areas. If you are bumped, check for your valuables.
- **AVOID** advertising where wallet is when you touch or fiddle with the pocket containing it. Try and keep wallet in inside front pocket.
- Be **AWARE** of travel wallets and money belts that are functional to offer better protection: RFID blocking products, and a retractable security metal spring loaded chain that anchors on wallet from pocket to belt.

June 12

ELEVATORS

- Be **ALERT** and **AWARE** by scanning the inside of the elevator before getting in. If you are alone and feel uncomfortable due to suspicious person(s), **AVOID** entering.
- Always try to stand near the control panel.
- Be **ALERT** and exit if someone suspicious enters.
- If you are attacked, press the alarm and as many of the control buttons as possible.
- Run your fingers up and down the floor buttons.
- Be **ALERT** for pickpockets on crowded elevators. Secure valuables.

June 13

JOGGING, WALKING

- Look and walk with confidence at a steady pace. Make eye contact with people.
- In public social situations, or when otherwise distracted (at the ATM, pumping gas into your vehicle), be **ALERT** and **AWARE of** keeping an eye on your surroundings. **AVOID** becoming so immersed in your activity that you lose touch with your surroundings and **ALERTNESS.**
- Confine these activities to daylight hours and to open, well-traveled areas. If you must run, walk, or jog at night, be **ALERT** to wear a reflective vest. Stay in well-lit areas.
- Wear a fanny pack to carry cell phone, keys.
- **AVOID** wearing shoes or clothing that restricts your movements.
- Be **AWARE**. Recognize your vulnerability and limitations.

June 14

- Be **ALERT** and **AWARE.**
- What is the landscape around you?
- Are you in a well-traveled area, or on a sparsely populated street, hidden from view?
- Are those around you walking with purpose, or are they just hanging around or watching others?
- **AVOID** shortcuts. Walking across an alley can put you in shadows and expose you to potential dangers of being attacked and robbed.
- **AVOID** hidden doorways, shrubs, and other areas where criminals may hide when stalking their prey.
- **AVOID** shortcuts, shrubbery, bushes, alleyways, or any other areas where an assailant might lurk or hide.
- **AVOID** athletic fields and tennis courts after dark.

NOTE:

In the United States, Flag Day is celebrated on June 14. It commemorates the adoption of the flag of the United States, which happened on that day in 1777, by resolution of the Second Continental Congress.

June 15

- Trust your gut feelings. If you feel something's not right, it probably isn't right.
- Confine walking to well-lit, regularly traveled walks and pathways.
- When returning to your vehicle or residence, have your keys, ready in hand in-between your fingers.
- Be **AWARE** of the panic alarm button on your car key fob if you are near your car.
- If threatened by an approaching vehicle, turn in the opposite direction or cross street.
- If you think you are being followed, cross the street, and if necessary, keep crossing back and forth. If you are pursued, yell for help, use cell phone, and run for aid.
- If someone suspicious passes you and turns a corner, be **ALERT** and **AWARE.**

June 16

PARKING

- Be **ALERT** and try to park in well-lit, busy areas.
- Be **ALERT** and **AVOID** parking between two vehicles that block your vehicle from the view of onlookers.
- **AVOID** leaving items of value, wallets, briefcases, packages, cell phones, computer bags in plain view. Place valuables in trunk BEFORE you get to your destination, not after. That's an opportunity for watchful thieves.

June 17

- In underground parking garages, be **ALERT** to park close to the entry/elevator.
- Be **ALERT** and try to park in an end spot for visibility.
- When there are times, you cannot leave valuables at home, or if your vehicle doesn't have a trunk (SUV, truck), be **ALERT** and place them on the floor or under seats. Shield them from open view.

<u>NOTE:</u>

Father's Day is celebrated in the US, Canada and the UK on the third Sunday in June. So, "Tie" one on safely!

June 18

PUBLIC TRANSPORTATION

Airplanes...

- **AVOID** packing expensive items in checked baggage. Take them in your carry-on luggage.
- **AVOID** leaving your luggage unattended, even for a brief moment, and be **AWARE** of distractions.
- Placing a band, strap, or tie around luggage, or a seal on the zipper, as an effective deterrent against theft.

Taxis...

- Note the driver's identification number.
- Be **ALERT** you are paying the right fare.
- Be **AWARE** of ghost or illegal taxis.
- Pre-book a taxi when traveling alone.

June 19

Trains, Buses, Subways...

- With careful planning, you might be able to **AVOID** long waits.
- When waiting, try and stay in populated areas, and if possible, in view of uniformed employees.
- Secure your personal belongings close to your body.
- **AVOID** displaying expensive jewelry, luggage, and briefcases.
- Are your valuables, such as computer, electronic devices etched with your ID? Do you have serial numbers, information on items if stolen for police reports?

June 20

SHOPPING

- After you have completed a purchase, be **ALERT** that you placed your cash, change, and all of your credit cards back in wallet before you leave counter.
- Check your receipts for corrections.
- Check that receipts do not show a full credit card number.
- **AVOID** overloading yourself with packages.
- Keep your arms and hands free.
- It is important to have clear visibility and freedom of motion when you are out. Dress comfortably.
- The more encumbered you are, the less you can move and escape.

"We used to build civilizations.
Now we build shopping malls."

~ BILL BRYSON

June 21

VEHICLE

- **AVOID** traveling on unknown roads.
- It is better to be safe than sorry by spending a few extra minutes to obtain travel directions and be **AWARE** of the best routes, best roads on a main highway.
- **AVOID** picking up hitchhikers or offering rides to strangers.
- Women suspects can and do attack lone drivers.
- If you pass a stranded motorist, even a woman, call the police and let them handle it.
- Police files are filled with examples of how good Samaritans have been victims of robbery or rape by supposedly stranded motorists or hitch hikers.
- A shortcut across an alley can put you in shadows and expose you to potential dangers of being attacked and robbed.
- Stay in well-lit areas during night hours.

June 22

- **AVOID** leaving valuables, briefcase, in your car and in plain view. Place them in the trunk.
- If your vehicle breaks down, call for help on the cell phone, lock all windows and doors on the vehicle, and don't open the vehicle for anyone until help arrives.
- Keep your car in good running condition, including tires (and spare), oil, water, battery.
- Be **ALERT, AWARE** there's enough gas to get where you're going and back (never let gas tank get less than one-quarter full).
- When stopped in traffic, always leave enough space between your car and one in front of you. This will allow you to pass easily if necessary and **AVOIDS** being sandwiched in as a potential robbery victim for these type of crimes.
- While driving, keep doors and windows locked to prevent a carjacking.

June 23

VIOLENCE PREVENTION FOR MEN

- Many men who survive violence are left with permanent physical and emotional scars. Violence can do terrible damage to a man's work, his health, his family, and his whole community.
- Men can, and have been, victims of intimate partner violence or domestic violence. They also feel uncomfortable reporting it.
- No one deserves to be hurt.
- If you have been emotionally, physically, or sexually abused, seek help. Talk with someone, whether a doctor, counselor, religious or community organization.
- You are not at fault.
- It is always wrong, whether the abuser is a family member, a current or past spouse, friend, or stranger.

June 24

Your best defense and offense strategies that can aid against becoming a victim are *The Unique Triple A*™ principles:

- Be **AWARE.** Eliminate potential dangers.
- Be **ALERT.** Recognize, and
- **AVOID** danger.

June 25

Today...

Give careful forethought to your own specific circumstances
and lifestyle. List five circumstances on how to **AVOID** a possible dangerous situation.

1. _____
   _____
   _____

2. _____
   _____
   _____

3. _____
   _____
   _____

4. _____
   _____
   _____

5. _____
   _____
   _____

June 26

- Don't think that it can't happen to you.
- Make yourself a "tough target."
- Should you resist? Every person and every situation is different.
- Always be **AWARE** of your surroundings.

June 27

In *The Unique Triple A™ Safety Handbook: How To Defend Yourself Without A Fight,* you will learn the 3 *Unique Triple A's*™ to crime prevention: **ALERT**, **AWARE,** and **AVOID.** Together, with the 3 P's of Prepare, Prevent and Protect, you have ingredients for a powerful mindset of confidence in dealing with potential dangerous and emergency situations.

- Learn to be **ALERT** to Prepare you, your family, your community, and home safer.
- Learn to be **AWARE** to Prevent yourself from being victimized.
- Learn to Protect, **AVOID** and refuse to be a victim.

June 28

TEACHABLE MOMENTS

Be a role model. Men – as fathers, brothers, coaches, teachers, uncles, and mentors – have a role to play in coaching boys into men.

Educate about honoring and respecting women, girls, and others. Show how to build attitudes and behaviors with young males to prevent relationship abuse. Share your own experiences and what you've learned.

You can do your part to stop violence by being a good role model to the young men in your life. Many young men want advice on how to deal with conflict and behave in relationships, but may not know how to ask for your help. You can make a real difference in boys' lives.

June 29

Studies have shown that involvement of a father or a positive male role model has profound effects on children.

How can you make a positive difference for these children?

Positive male role models can get involved in and influence the lives of children in their communities.

Non-custodial dads can make the effort to visit with their children more often and teach them important life lessons.

Educators can encourage fathers to take on a more active role in the school their kids attend.

Faith-based institutions can provide programs for fathers and sons and encourage male role models.

Business leaders can encourage employees to be involved in community efforts such as mentoring and youth groups.

June 30

HEALTH AND STRESS MANAGEMENT

Adults, teens, and even children experience stress at times. Stress can sometimes be beneficial by helping develop skills needed to cope with, and adapt to, new and potentially threatening situations throughout life. Yet, beneficial aspects can diminish when it is severe enough to overwhelm a person's ability to take care of themselves and/or family. Use healthy ways to cope, and obtain the right care and support to put issues in perspective and help you gain control of your life and take care of your family.

- Take care of yourself. Eat healthy, well-balanced meals. Exercise on a regular basis.
- Get plenty of sleep.
- Give yourself a break if you feel stressed out, especially from everyday life.
- Talk to others, professionals. Share your problems, and how you are feeling and coping, depressed, or thinking about suicide.

BONUS SAFETY TIP

Shift the odds to your favor. Minimize opportunity for trouble by recognizing that the best defense against crime is to prevent it from ever occurring. Common sense and crime prevention are the best tools available. Think of "supply and demand." The supply is bounteous. Almost everyone carries a purse or wallet, or is vulnerable. The demand for easy access to them and valuables equals or exceeds the supply. Without *The Unique Triple A*™ you have the perfect supply and demand formula for crime and victims.

It is time to stop living in denial and depending on police to protect you and your family 24 hours. Take action. Your safety is your responsibility and up to you to either get trained in self-defense classes, or be **AWARE** of your vulnerabilities and do something about them. It's your choice.

"Thought is action in rehearsal."

~ RALPH WALDO EMERSON

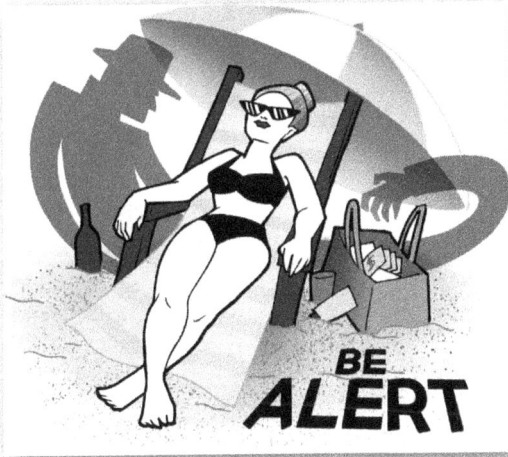

BE
ALERT

July

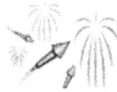

FIRECRACKER TIPS

Hit The Road Jack

July 1

PLANNING AHEAD SAFER VACATIONS

- **AVOID** sharing and broadcasting vacation plans on social networking and other sites.

- Secure ladders and tools so they can't be used to gain entry into your home. Put items such as lawn furniture and bicycles away before leaving, as items left out can easily be stolen. Be **ALERT** and **AWARE** you have good locks on all doors and windows. Repair broken windows and screens, and insure all doors and window locks function and lock securely. When you leave be **ALERT** that your back door and windows are locked securely.

- Contact a neighbor or relative to pick up or throw away papers, solicitation notices, and any delivered packages. Hold the delivery of mail and newspapers. Be **AWARE** that post offices offer to place mail on "vacation hold."

- Be **AWARE** that your smoke and burglar alarms function and are armed properly.

July 2

- Be **ALERT** to maintain that "lived in" look by lowering the ring on your phone and arranging a trusted friend, relative, or neighbor do some yard work upkeep or occasionally park a car in your driveway.

- Leave the shades and blinds on doors and windows in a position that you would normally have them, but not completely open. Use timers for lights, television, or radio to make the house appear as if it's currently occupied. Set them in a random pattern.

- In packing, be **ALERT** that you may lose stuff. Plan and be **ALERT** not to pack anything that you could not bear to part with, especially sentimental or valuable items. Pack key items in your carry-on bag like extra underwear or essential items for a business meeting so you can continue your trip if your checked bags are lost or delayed.

- Carry small denominations of cash for tips at restaurants, cruise ships, hotels, etc.

July 3

CELEBRATORY FIREARMS SHOOTING

Enjoy Independence Day, but check your area if fireworks possession/use are legal. Refer to local fire department for firework safety and proper use of fire extinguishers. Parents must be responsible to ensure their weapons are locked securely and unreachable from family household members.

On holidays, such as 4th of July and New Year's Eve, irresponsible persons shoot off firearms to "celebrate," and at times, begin before the holiday and continue for the next couple of days thereafter. This is a dangerous and illegal practice that has caused death and injuries every year from stray bullets that go up into the air and speed down at terminal velocity. A small-caliber bullet can travel up to two miles into the air and pick up enough speed to crash through a human skull or a house roof. This is a crime punishable by law, and if a bullet is found to have killed someone, the person responsible may be prosecuted for murder. Anyone who sees someone fire a gun in the air is asked to call 9-1-1.

July 4

Public Displays...

Dress kids in bright colors to recognize in crowded areas (if separated), when you attend public fireworks displays. Stay behind safety barriers. Parents, accompany and supervise children in public facilities, including restrooms.

Fire Extinguishers...

- Select correct extinguishers.
- Use properly.
- Join a local fire department C.E.R.T. class.

NOTE:

How Well Do You Know The Star Spangled Banner?

Which US president signed the law designating it as the national anthem?

    a.   Calvin Coolidge
    b.   Warren G. Harding
    c.   Herbert Hoover
    d.   Franklin D. Roosevelt

You look up the answer and source this time.

July 5

PLANNING AHEAD SAFER VACATIONS

Be **AWARE** of your expensive items, such as jewelry, and **AVOID** expensive jewelry or other valuables being taken while you are away.

- Open a safety deposit box at your bank. Be **ALERT** that keeping valuables in a safety deposit box is the best permanent option.
- Consider what jewelry to wear during your vacation, and ask yourself if it is flashy, expensive, or looks expensive. Better yet, **AVOID** traveling with valuables you do not want to lose.
- Necklaces, for example, are easy to "snatch and grab" as the chains break easily.
- Check with hotel staff you made reservations with for recommendations.
- When researching or making hotel reservations, be **AWARE** to inquire about hotel safes at the desk and/or in rooms.

July 6

- Be **AWARE** and be travel SMART. Set up a special travel account and credit card not linked to your checking and savings accounts. Deposit only the money you want to spend and use that credit card during your trip. Credit cards have greater protection against fraudulent activity, liability losses.

- Plan ahead and consider where you're going, and what you'll be doing. Be **ALERT** and **AWARE** to learn about your vacation destination before you arrive; know what sites you want to visit and how to get there using a safe, well-traveled route. When traveling, always be **ALERT** to your surroundings and know how to reach your destinations prior to your departure.

- **AVOID** carrying more cash and credit cards than you will need. Use traveler's checks and carry only cash and credit cards you plan and need. Keep a list of toll-free numbers when needed.

July 7

- Stay **AWARE** and **ALERT** to vacation rental scams. Con artists do place phony ads at great prices.
- Con artists steal property descriptions and photos listed on legitimate real estate websites or post addresses of homes that are not for rent.
- They often show up on Craigslist, newspapers, chat boards, phony real estate websites that they create.
- Be **ALERT** they will ask for up-front payment or personal information to steal your identity.
- Be **ALERT** to check out the property yourself, online, or with a legitimate realtor.
- Use search engine to obtain an aerial view of the property.
- Select sightseeing companies and guides carefully. Make sure they are legitimate.

July 8

Togetherness...

Finding airline seats together, especially for small children or family member with special needs is not easy unless you pay more. Things you can try:

- Book as far ahead as possible. Speak to the airline to see if representatives will open up adjacent seats.
- Enter your child's age when making a reservation.
- Get to the airport very early and speak to the check-in agent. You might be able to snag some seats held back for elite-status passengers.
- Change plans or airlines. Choose flights offering seats together, even if it means changing plans or buying more expensive seats.
- At time of writing, check with airlines, such as Southwest Airlines, that may still offer priority boarding to parents with kids under 4 and those with needs.

July 9

TRAVEL INSURANCE

- Be **ALERT** and **AWARE** you understand the right level of travel insurance, such as luggage and medical emergency, especially in a foreign country.
- Read the policy description thoroughly and be **AWARE** of any policy regarding valuable items and/or full coverage.
- Check with your insurance company if you have travel insurance and what it covers or does not cover.

July 10

IMMUNIZATIONS

- Be **AWARE** when making travel plans out of the country to research phone numbers/addresses to the U.S. embassy in case an emergency situation arises.

- Be **AWARE** if booster shots are required. Are you also **AWARE** of your blood type, and if passport is in order?

- When traveling to international countries, be **ALERT** to consult a travel health specialist or the World Health Organization (WHO), concerning immunizations and requirements to your destinations and specific itinerary. Your immunizations should be documented in an International Certificate of Vaccination (Yellow Card). Make a copy and keep this certificate with your passport so you don't misplace it as it is recognized internationally.

- May be required before entry to certain countries, or re-entry into the US. Decisions based on geographic area, purpose, and duration of travel, and the anticipated level of contact with the local population.

July 11

Pet Vaccinations...

Take pets to a vet no less than two weeks before departing for fleas/tick preventatives, micro-chipping, physical and/or required vaccinations. Ensure all vaccinations/prescriptions are current.

If your pet needs a procedure, schedule it early for recovery to reduce the likelihood of a pricey overnight stay.

Pet SMART...

Be **AWARE** that ASPCA recommends feeding at least three hours before departure, and cautions against feeding a pet inside a moving vehicle and sticking head out of moving car windows (susceptible to ear and lung infections). Use a crate or carrier to prevent injury in a collision. Also acts as a familiar bed in an unfamiliar location. Take medications, first aid kit, grooming supplies, towels, waste scooper, food/water bowls, toys, etc.

Compare and save costs on meds at sites like http://www. PetCareRX.com, or 1.800.PetMeds.

July 12

LUGGAGE SAFETY

- Mark your luggage so it is easily identified.
- Take photos so airline personnel can identify it if it is lost.
- Be **AWARE** to consider purchasing a pack of plastic zip ties (or cable locks), in different colors to use as double safety with your locks, as these are useful for making sure your bags are not tampered with in hotel, or airport, or if your luggage was opened or inspected by TSA.
- Mix up the colors for additional security.
- If your bag appears on an airport carousel with the cable ties missing, or the color combination changed, don't touch the bag, but call security and advise of possible tampering or theft.
- Always check contents before you leave the airport.
- Be **ALERT** your luggage is locked and labeled with your name and telephone number. Use alternate number, such as office or P.O. Box.

July 13

- Use tags of metal, plastic, or leather as paper tags get wet or damaged.
- Be **ALERT** that airline personnel may insist on checking larger carry-on bags if the overhead bins become filled.
- Be **AWARE** and plan how much gear and luggage you really need.
- Be **AWARE** it is much easier to get around with less luggage. You are more **ALERT** in keeping track and an eye on fewer bags than too many.
- Be **ALERT** to place an emergency supply kit in your carry-on. Be **AWARE** when packing to carry extra medication, prescriptions, lenses/glasses, or anything you will need in an emergency if lost, stolen.
- If traveling by car, include seat belt cutters.
- Be **ALERT** for shorter trips and travel with only a carry-on.

July 14

- By using carry-on luggage, you are less apt of having it lost or stolen. But, be **ALERT** to your carry-ons.
- Be **ALERT** to check baggage charges on all airlines and purchase a portable digital luggage weighing scale to **AVOID** overweight baggage fees. Review http://www. AirSafe.com information for general baggage resources for general limits on carry-on luggage.
- Be **ALERT** to keep the stub from your checked luggage in a safe, secure place. This critical document is needed if your luggage is lost. You will need proof that you own the luggage.
- Immediately report any loss or theft of luggage.
- Money, laptop computers, electronic files, and other items of high value or importance should be kept in a carry-on bag that can also stow under a seat.
- **AVOID** leaving luggage alone for even a minute at car rentals, airports, restaurants. Never leave unattended, keep in sight.

July 15

- Thieves can act with extraordinary rapidity and your bag can vanish or have stuff selectively swiped from it in the blink of an eye.

- Always be **AWARE** and **ALERT** that the airline tag on your checked luggage is for the correct destination.

- Be **AWARE** of luggage contents when crossing borders, catching flights, or passing through customs.

- **AVOID** offering to carry anything for anyone else but your family.

- Be **AWARE** you are not importing illegal substances, which could be as innocent as fruit or alcohol, as fines or even jail may be imposed.

- Every piece of checked luggage should have a three-letter airport identifier that matches your destination airport.

- If you are unsure of the code, ask the ticket agent or skycap.

July 16

CAR RENTALS

- Be **ALERT** and **AWARE** of car rental scams.
- **AVOID** responding to ads and use legitimate business rentals.
- **ALERT** yourself to the vehicle's safety equipment, including hazard lights, windshield wipers, spare tire, seat belts, and door locks.
- Be **ALERT** and review maps and other visitor information and how to reach your destinations before leaving the rental car area.
- **AVOID** leaving luggage unattended for even a minute at car rentals, airports, restaurants. If there is more than one person in your party, assign someone to stay with the bags.
- Check with ACRA (American Car Rental Association), to confirm that the car rental business is a registered one.

July 17

Car Security Rentals...

- Thieves target rental cars that look like rental cars (company name on license frame).
- **AVOID** leaving rental indicators (maps, rental paperwork, agreement, even your luggage), in plain view.
- **AVOID** leaving valuables, purses, briefcases, important papers in plain view.
- Be **AWARE** all doors and windows are locked and secured before entering and exiting.
- Park in well-lighted areas or as close to the front of the hotel as possible, especially after dark.
- **AVOID** leaving the car running unattended, even to dash into a store.
- Be **ALERT** and **AWARE** gas tank is always full and the locations of gas stations. Check your phone apps for locations.

July 18

Tire SMART...

- Maintenance. Schedule for wheel alignment and rotation about every 5,000 to 8,000 miles. Check owner's manual.

- Tire pressure gauge. Recommended tire pressure is on a sticker on driver's side doorjamb, or in vehicle owner's manual, or inside gas cap door. Do not refer to numbers on tires.

- Tread-depth gauge measures remaining tread on tires. Near the 2/32-inch mark is time to replace them.

- Regularly check tire sidewalls for gouges or other damage, and nails in tread.

- Timely maintenance can head off costly repairs and inconveniences on the road. Tires low of air pose safety risks, waste fuel, and can self-destruct.

- Check your owner's manual for scheduled brake pad maintenance.

July 19

CASH, CREDIT CARDS, CELL PHONES

- The best way to keep valuables safe while traveling is to **AVOID** bringing them at all.
- If you do, before you reserve hotel or cruise ship rooms, ask manager about their security systems.
- Be **AWARE** of the security of room safes. Reported police cases reveal maids or employees getting into them and removing items.
- Take only one or two credit cards widely used. **AVOID** letting your card out of your sight or anyone, such as a salesclerk or waiter, walk off with your card.
- Contact your credit card companies and bank to advise you will be using them, and the dates and locations of your travels.
- Ascertain how to report a lost or stolen card before you leave, and retain card contact numbers. Keep all receipts
- **AVOID** carrying large amounts of cash (small denominations). Carry only the credit cards or cash needed for that day.
- Be **AWARE** of duplicate charges on cards.

July 20

- When traveling abroad, be **AWARE** to ascertain accepted appropriate credit cards to the countries of your destinations, ATM cash and card withdrawal limits (including 24-hour period), fees (currency exchanges and transactions).

- Stay **AWARE** and keep a list of important financial numbers.

- Be careful what you say on financial, travel plans. Cell phone interception is one of the easiest ways to steal information. How does it work? An interceptor gets between the targeted phone and the network tower, fooling your phone into thinking it's an actual tower. But, the interceptor doesn't look like a tower. It's more like the size of a briefcase or a laptop.

July 21

Credit Cards

- Company _____

- Number to call if lost/stolen _____

Traveler's Checks

- Numbers _____

- If lost/stolen, call _____

Other Useful Numbers

- Physician _____

- Prescription numbers _____

July 22

TIPS AT THE AIRLINE SECURITY CHECKS

Be **AWARE** and **ALERT** not to be a forgetful traveler. Transportation Security Administration (TSA), lost-and-found offices have turned into digital treasure troves because most people forget to retrieve their items after going through checkpoints, or forgot where they lost the items while in transit (taxi cabs, shuttles, restaurants, hotels). Unclaimed items officially become the property of the federal government after 30 days. Though TSA workers will attempt to try and find contact information, other than passports and driver's license, most items collected are not reclaimed.

- Tape a business card to all valuable electronics.
- Put small items (wallet, keys, phones), in carry-on bag before passing through security. You may not need to take off small pieces of jewelry for the metal detector. Be **ALERT** and don't rush through checkpoints. Pay attention.

July 23

DINING OUT

- Stay **ALERT** to distractions or anyone you don't know.
- Be **ALERT** and keep purse on lap.
- Straps on luggage can be slipped around your chair leg and bags under table.
- Separate your money, passport, valuables from luggage.
- Be **ALERT** and **AWARE** to pay for your dining purchases at the register. **AVOID** handing card to waiter at table. It's not unheard of to have a restaurant worker walk away and scam your card. It's also not unheard of, other than your server, to collect the check, or someone who is not an employee to pose as a "waiter" and take your check. Then again, legitimate restaurant employees have been known to commit fraud with a patron's credit card, because it's customary that servers will take your card out of sight, providing an opportunity to copy the information.

July 24

HEAT EXHAUSTION AND STRESS

- Be **AWARE** that physical activity at high temperatures can directly affect your health.
- Discomfort includes cramps, weakness, headaches, and dizziness. Can result in convulsions, unconsciousness, coma, or death.
- Be **AWARE** to drink water or potassium, sodium replacement-type liquids every 15-30 minutes.
- Dress sensibly and wear light-colored, cotton clothing, keep shirt on.
- Be **ALERT** to drink plenty of water. Stay hydrated.
- **AVOID** heavy meals. Eat lightly.

July 25

HOTELS AND MOTELS

- Place all your luggage in your room.
- Unpack your luggage and arrange all your belongings so that you will notice if anything is missing. Keep a daily check of all your belongings. **AVOID** leaving valuables in your room when you are not there. Check to see if the bank you use is in the places you are in. Ask your bank if they would allow a courtesy safety deposit box for your items.
- Place extra cash, jewelry, or valuables in a hotel/motel safe. **AVOID** flashing your cash.
- Use the door viewer to identify anyone requesting entry into your room. **AVOID** opening the door if you do not believe the person has a legitimate reason for being in your room.
- While staying in a hotel room, be **ALERT** to familiarize yourself with the door locks, emergency exits, and other safety features.
- **AVOID** leaving any tickets (airline, train, bus) in open view (poolside).

July 26

PASSPORTS, WI-FI NETWORKS

Make a copy of passport and keep separate from credit cards. Always present the photocopy first. **AVOID** putting anything important in your pockets, wallets, purses, or bags that your carry. Place them in a money belt or secret pocket.

Be **ALERT** when searching for Wi-Fi networks. Be **ALERT** when using any public network, that it is fully encrypted and **AVOID** using the same password on different websites. Be **AWARE** and change your mobile device settings to **AVOID** automatic connection to a nearby Wi-Fi network. **AVOID** online banking. Be **ALERT** that public Wi-Fi is shared. If a public Wi-Fi hotspot doesn't require a WPA or WPA2 password, it's not secure. Choose apps wisely. Before downloading an app, check the app's security policies. What information does it collect, and how will it protect data during transmission and storage?

Confirm hotel authorized network before you connect.

July 27

PUBLIC TRANSPORTATION

- Be **AWARE** of any foreign countries that require luggage to be placed on bus roofs.
- Carry your valuables on your person or carry-on. **AVOID** leaving carry-on unattended.
- Be **ALERT** and **AWARE** when exiting that you have all your luggage/belongings with you.
- Be **ALERT** and **AWARE** of potential pickpockets, and where you placed your wallet, and how you carry your purse. Use a fanny pack.
- When asking for directions, first look for a police officer or another public employee (bus driver), or go into a nearby business.
- Don't advertise that you're a tourist by leaving maps and guidebooks on a car seat or dashboard. Keep them in the glove compartment.

July 28

RECREATIONAL SAFETY

Hiking, Walking...

AVOID cotton socks in favor of moisture-wicking nylon or acrylic to keep feet dry. Use petroleum jelly or *Body Glide* to help prevent blisters. Layer by wearing a light windbreaker or jacket during the cooler morning; tie it around your waist when it warms up. Use a fanny pack for food, water, keys, ID, sunscreen, and first aid supplies. Eat a healthy breakfast like oatmeal or yogurt.

Basics should include a charged cell phone, GPS device, water, maps of area, compass, extra clothing and food, first aid kit, pocket knife. Poison oak is identified by its three leaves. Until you can seek medical attention, **AVOID** scratching and try to apply cold water and cloth compress for relief. Aloe or an over-the-counter product containing bentoquatam soothes. Bring the appropriate medicines for allergies and allergies to bee stings.

Stay on known trails and let someone know where you will be.

July 29

SIGHT-SEEING

- Be **ALERT** and plan ahead.
- Ask for directions and safety tips at a hotel/motel on how to get to attractions you want to visit.
- Ask if there are any areas in town you should **AVOID**.
- Stay **ALERT** and stick to well-lighted main streets and public areas.
- **AVOID** looking lost (stopping and looking at addresses or street signs).
- Go to an open business if you feel you are lost.

Make A Map From Your Photos...

http://www.urbanbird.io creates a map from the photos you upload and captions them with dates, location, titles, and descriptions. Make sure your camera or smartphone are set to geotag your photos before you start snapping your pictures. The site is working on adding comments manually.

July 30

WATER SAFETY

Be **ALERT** and **AWARE** where children are near water, such as water parks, lakes, oceans, or pools.

Number of drowning deaths by age: 1 year 2%; 1-3 years 64%; 4 years 11%; 5-9 years 17%, and 10-14 years 5% with CA, AZ, FL, and TX as leading states (U.S. Consumer Product Safety Commission or http://www.cpsc.gov).

Does the pool or spa use appropriate water safety practices, barriers, safety covers, fences, appropriate equipment, (safety drain covers, life rings, reaching poles available)? Lifeguard or sufficient staff at pool, ocean? Do you or your children know how to swim? Know CPR? Are you **ALERT, AWARE,** in watching your children?

Be **ALERT** to hazardous weather advisories/warnings on high surf and strong rip currents.

July 31

THE RESPONSIBLE VACATION TRAVELER

Travel and tourism supports jobs worldwide and generates a percentage of the world's gross domestic product. It's important to leave a positive impact and to travel in a way that doesn't change the places and people you visit in a negative way.

Every year, http://www.ethicaltraveler.org reviews the policies and practices of scores of nations in the developing world that do the most impressive job of promoting human rights, preserving their environments, and supporting social welfare – all while creating a lively, community-based tourism industry. By visiting these countries, you use your economic leverage as travelers to support best practices. People who travel can feel a sense of stewardship for the world. Explore these destinations and enjoy the sights, cultures, and inspirations they offer.

Patronize locally-owned inns, restaurants, shops. Le-ave hotel rooms clean when you leave. Be courteous.

BONUS SAFETY TIP

Travel Smart, Reduce Health And Safety Risks...

Suggested items for traveling, whether by car or other:

Automatic cordless tire inflator, no-blind spot rearview mirror, portable luggage weight scale, RFID blocking credit card protector, dry stick spot cleaner, travel neck pillow, motion-sickness product, flight nasal spray-all natural antibacterial/anti-fungal product, hanging toiletry kit organizer, bed bug travel luggage spray, TSA compliant bottle travel set.

Be **ALERT, AWARE** you and your passengers wear seat belts, and **AWARE** of child passenger safety restraint seat requirements (http://www.nhtsa.gov).

Be **AWARE** to protect back with selected luggage. Look for sturdy, light, high-quality, transportable pieces with wheels, handle, not heavy/bulky.

To lift luggage: stand alongside of it, bend at knees, limit bending at the waist, lift luggage with leg muscles, grasp handle, and straighten up. Once you lift the luggage, hold it close to your body.

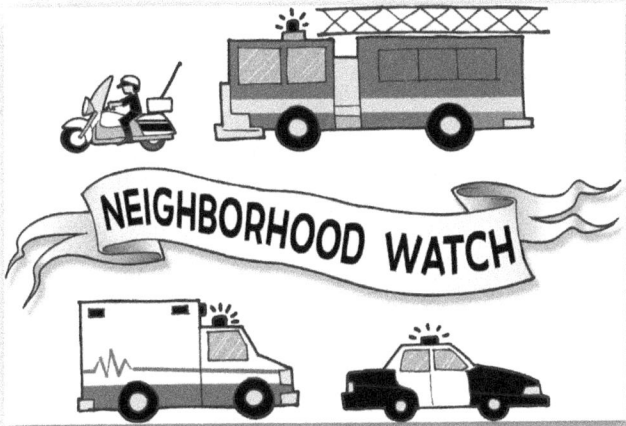

August

NATIONAL NITE OUT

Home & Community

August 1

WHAT IS NATIONAL NITE OUT?

It's a community event celebrated annually since 1984 on the first Tuesday in August throughout the US and Canada with a focus on strengthening neighborhoods and preventing crime. It is sponsored by the National Association of Town Watch in the US and Canada.

National Night Out is designed to heighten crime prevention **AWARENESS**, generate support for, and participation in, local anti-crime efforts, strengthen neighborhood spirit in the crime prevention campaign, and send a message to criminals to let them know neighborhoods are organized and fighting back. The event is meant to increase **AWARENESS** about police programs in communities, such as drug prevention, Town Watch, or Neighborhood Watch, and other anti-crime efforts, such as burglary, gangs, and violence.

August 2

- Neighborhoods can heighten community awareness of gangs, crime, and drug prevention.
- Generate support for, and participation in, local anti-crime programs with law enforcement.
- Sends a message to criminals that neighborhoods are organized and fighting back.
- Promotes emergency preparedness **AWARE-NESS.**
- Strengthens neighborhood spirit and police-community partnership in order to help prevent or **AVOID** crime.
- Get to know your neighbors so you can work together and look out for each other if there is any suspicious behavior happening in your neighborhood.
- Identify vital elements for starting and maintaining community mobilization efforts, and look at surmounting common obstacles.

August 3

HOW DO NEIGHBORS PARTICIPATE?

The events are typically organized by block watches, non-for-profit organizations, companies, and law enforcement agencies. These events can be as simple as neighborhood cookouts to full-blown festivals, parades, live music, food, entertainment, or whatever brings people out to get involved in anti-crime efforts.

Receive assistance from local police department to organize a Neighborhood Watch regarding gangs and crime prevention, and learn to be **ALERT, AWARE,** and **AVOID.**

Work with neighbors, local government businesses, civic groups, and individuals, devoted to safer communities.

Organize community clean-ups. The cleaner your neighborhood, the less attractive it is to crime. Publish a neighborhood newsletter on local crime and crime prevention tips.

August 4

On the first Tuesday in August, everyone participates in National Nite Out by turning on their front porch lights to send a message to criminals, "not in our neighborhood." This traditional "lights on" campaign is a National Nite Out symbolic front porch vigil celebrated across America with various events and activities, such as block parties, cookouts, parades, visits from emergency personnel, rallies and marches, exhibits, youth events, safety demonstrations and seminars, in effort to heighten **AWARENESS** and enhance community relations.

National Nite Out celebrates safety and crime prevention successes, and works to expand and strengthen programs for 365 days.

*"An ounce of prevention is
worth a pound of cure."*

~ BENJAMIN FRANKLIN

August 5

WHAT IS NEIGHBORHOOD WATCH?

- An organized group of citizens devoted to crime and vandalism prevention within a community or neighborhood.
- Neighbors keep an **ALERT** eye on one another's properties and report suspicious incidents to the police.
- Your local police department will assist to help set up a Neighborhood Watch, distribute handouts, and instruct how to order Neighborhood Watch warning decals and street signs.
- Below, list the phone number and contact at your local police agency for more information.

August 6

HOME

Check Outside Perimeter Of Your Home...

- Stay **ALERT** and **AWARE.** Stand in front of your home, analyze its weaknesses and strengths the way a criminal or burglar would.

- First, keep your yard clean. Prune back shrubbery in front of, or near, doors and windows to **AVOID** hiding places and concealment for criminals. Trim shrubs below windowsill at least 5 inches above ground to **AVOID** concealment.

- Plant hardy, fast-growing and thorny bushes or vines as an extra barrier around the perimeter.

- Check with your local garden nursery for thorny shrubbery.

- Trim out tree leaves and cut back tree limbs away from upper-level windows and roof to eliminate entry and hiding spots.

- Consider installing a gravel path near bedroom windows to **ALERT** you to a prowler.

August 7

- Install a secure fence to deter someone access to your home and through your back door.
- Help **AVOID** crime opportunities. Remove ladders, trash bins, or other objects thieves can and will use to climb to an upper-level area.
- Install reflective address numbers in a visible location, front and back, so emergency personnel can locate your home quickly.
- Be **ALERT** to secure all outdoor and personal property such as bikes (place in garage), grills, lawn mowers, patio furniture, and pool gates, with quality cable locks, u-locks, and padlocks to prevent theft.

August 8

Doors And Windows...

- **AVOID** hollow core doors on all doors, including rear doors, and replace with metal or solid core wooden doors.
- If your doors do not fit tightly in their frames, install weather stripping around them.
- If your doors have conventional glass panels, (how close is glass to inside door lock?) consider replacing them with shatterproof glass or with polycarbonate material.
- A simple, inexpensive safety device is a one-way door viewer for **AWARENESS**.
- Burglar-proof your glass patio doors by setting a pipe or metal bar/rod in the middle bottom track of the door slide. The pipe should be the same length as the track.
- Install and use deadbolt locks on exterior doors that lead into the garage.
- Install parameter motion detectors for outdoors and inside home.

August 9

Locks...

- Locks should have deadbolts with full one-inch bolts on all entry doors.
- Be **ALERT** that these should be installed on front, back, and side doors in addition to existing locksets.
- Replace outdoor locks with Grade-1 double- cylinder deadbolts with at least two one-quarter-inch case hardened bolts equipped with a cylinder guard to prevent vice-grip type tools used in turning or breaking lock.
- Are you **AWARE** that deadbolts should be placed at least 12 inches above the doorknob and at least 40 inches away from windows, glass panels, and other openings such as mail slots (**AVOID** placement near inside locks)?

August 10

- The strike plate should consist of heavy-gauge metal with four screws, minimum of 3-inches long.
- Digital locks include pushbutton locks, fingerprint locks, and remote-controlled locks.
- Be **AWARE** when choosing digital home locks to be sure there is no keyhole (easy to lock pick).
- Be **ALERT** to closely inspect deadbolts every six months for tampering and excess wear.

August 11

Garage...

- Garage doors should have devices that prevent forced entry, such as sensors, automatic lights, locking mechanisms, or reverse-opening capabilities.
- Should have safety features that reduce the risk of injury and fire.
- Ensure that doors inside the garage that lead to your house are of solid wood and locked securely at all times.
- Be **AWARE** that polyurethane-insulated door types have a higher R-value, which means they have better insulation properties.
- Install a secondary lock on the garage door and be **AWARE** not to count on the automatic garage door opener for security.
- Every bicycle in the garage should be secured with a U-bar lock, or quality padlock and chain.
- Be **ALERT** to secure ladders, tools and toolbox.

August 12

- Be **ALERT** and **AWARE** to keep garage doors closed at all times to safeguard your belongings and family.

- **AVOID** leaving the garage door open unattended even for a short period.

- Always be **AWARE** the garage interior door that gains entry to your house is locked and secured, especially when you are outside.

- Be **AWARE** that home security system components, such as an overhead garage door contact, can also provide added protection to your home.

- List contact information on the business that installed your garage door.

August 13

Lighting...

- Five practical crime prevention functions of lighting include; detection, deterrence, fear reduction, liability reduction, and surveillance.
- Lighting for homes and garages should focus on deterring criminals and providing surveillance opportunities for law enforcement, home residents, and neighbors.
- Be **ALERT** that badly designed lighting makes things better for criminals.
- Be **AWARE** that even well-applied illumination, is not always a cure-all preventative against crime ALONE.
- Prior to application and installation of fixtures, proper application and the right fixtures need to be analyzed for effectiveness.

August 14

- Be **ALERT** to ask questions about lighting security to assist you when choosing a professional.
- Is it cost effective? Are there less costly solutions?
- How would lighting help to reduce the crime or the risk of crime?
- How would outdoor motion lights work for your home? When installed, be **AWARE** that they can be seen from the street when they are activated.
- Will the lighting cause glare, distraction, or disruption (in their bedroom), to neighbors?
- What are you trying to create?

August 15

ALARM AND FIRE SYSTEMS

Home security system sensors help protect you from threats such as fire, carbon monoxide, flooding, home invasion, medical emergencies.

Always keep the correct fire extinguisher in easy-to reach locations and be **AWARE** that everyone knows how to properly use them. Contact your local fire department for appropriate extinguishers and usage.

Locate a Community Emergency Response Team (C.E.R.T.) fire department program by zip code and inquire about disaster training and volunteer opportunities near you.

Most alarm, cable, and satellite companies now offer a smart home surveillance system that you can keep track of your home with the use of your cell phone or computer, even when you are not there.

Be **ALERT** to change batteries on carbon monoxide and smoke alarms during time changes.

August 16

BURGLAR AND FIRE ESCAPE PLANS

- Be **ALERT** and involve entire household in planning what to do during a fire or burglary.

- Draw a floor plan of your house, rooms, hallways, doors, windows, exit points.

- Identify a meeting place outside home or neighborhood.

- Be **ALERT** to identify at least two exits from each room.

- Invest in a glass break sensor. When a glass door or window is shattered, the sensor will **ALERT** you of a break-in.

- For second or more story windows, have a fire escape ladder available in each room.

- Go over and walk through your plan, make a list of anything you need to purchase and install, and practice the "what ifs" so everyone understands and knows their roles.

- Get involved with neighbors, fire, and police on emergency preparedness.

August 17

- Have a fire extinguisher in garage and throughout house. Check with local fire department on correct extinguishers and how to use them properly. Sign up for C.E.R.T. courses (see GLOSSARY).
- Be **ALERT** and always lock your doors and windows when you are not at home, day and night.
- When you are home and wish to leave window(s) open, be **ALERT** to install safety latches or sliding door rods to **AVOID** windows that would open enough to allow unauthorized entry.
- **AVOID** leaving notes on the door when going out.
- When leaving for an extended period of time (days or weeks), notify the police and a neighbor, leave emergency contact information, who is allowed to be at the house, and what vehicles, if any, will be parked there.

August 18

- **AVOID** hiding spare keys under the doormat, mailbox, flowerpot, or in conspicuous places.
- Change your codes on security alarms, keyless entry doors, garage doors, and remote controls often.
- If you must leave your vehicle outside, be **ALERT** and **AWARE** that it is locked and there are no valuables inside.
- Park your vehicle in a well-lit area.
- Take the garage door opener and car keys with you instead of leaving in the vehicle.
- Be **AWARE** you can also use your car remote key to press the panic button for help. This will activate the car alarm, alerting neighbors and the intruder.

August 19

- **AVOID** keeping large amounts of cash or expensive jewelry around the house.
- Consider having a bank safety deposit box.
- Be **AWARE** of engraving tools that can mark or etch appropriate valuables with identification numbers.
- Videotape contents of your home, valuables, and jewelry.
- Keep an updated inventory list and photos/videos in a home safe or a bank safety deposit box.
- It's a good idea to keep backups of list in a secure, separate location as well.

August 20

CHILDPROOFING

- Install hardware-mounted secure safety gates at the top and bottom of stairways, or on doors that open into a stairway, to prevent fall-related injuries.
- Install a childproof lock on medicine cabinets.
- Consider using doorknob protectors.
- Be **ALERT** that doors to walk-in closets and pantries should open from the inside as well as the outside.
- **AVOID** and eliminate the loop in two-corded blinds and shades. Install a cord tie-down device to prevent children wrapping themselves around cords and prevent strangulation.

August 21

- Install outlet covers, outlet plugs, and plug locks on all outlets and cords currently not in use.
- **AVOID** thick pile carpeting, if at all possible. Small objects, such as buttons and sewing needles, can hide within the pile, easily finding their way to your child's mouth.
- Opt for tightly-woven, flat-weave, or low-pile carpeting.

August 22

FIREARMS

- Be **ALERT** and **AWARE** to ALWAYS keep guns unloaded and locked securely with bore, trigger, and/or slide locks.

- Must be unreachable by children or other untrained member of the household. Inquire with local law enforcement on safe storage and gun locks. Lock and store bullets in a separate location. Ensure children NEVER have access to the keys.

- Be **ALERT** and **AWARE** of all laws and/or firearm permits, and/or safety training courses where you reside and travel.

- Kids are curious. Talk with your children about the risks of firearms and to never touch a gun where they may visit or play.

- Check with local target ranges and law enforcement for training and education courses.

August 23

PANIC ROOMS

A panic room is a safe room used when unable to escape safely from an intruder or an emergency. Mostly installed in a main bedroom. Hide the panic door in a closet or behind a bookcase.

- Be **AWARE** to install a solid wood door, good deadbolts. Outfit room with cell phone with a guaranteed signal attachment, or a phone line, or ham radio, fire extinguisher, first aid kit, flashlights, battery-powered radio and batteries, non-perishable food, water, RV or composting toilet, locked and secured firearms.
- Reinforce walls with Kevlar, sheets of steel or bulletproof fiberglass. Soundproof walls to **AVOID** intruders from hearing you Install small videos around your home with a monitor in the safe room.

August 24

- Provide electricity and ventilation with a generator if the room will be used for several days.
- **AVOID** a generator in an unventilated room.
- Be **ALERT** to occasionally test flashlights, radio, phones, generator to ensure they are working.
- Rotate food if it passes expiration date. The Red Cross recommends one gallon of water per person per day.
- Be **ALERT** to have extra blankets, clothing, pillows in case of an extended stay.
- Stocks books, games, puzzles, magazines.
- Have a portable DVD player with charged batteries for children.

Under any circumstances, AVOID confronting a burglar. Initiate your emergency plan and leave the house immediately. Go to neighbor's home and call the police.

August 25

SOLICITORS

- **AVOID** solicitors so you won't have to be bothered.
- Be **ALERT** to ask to see their permit and their credentials along with a photo ID but **AVOID** opening door.
- Be **AWARE** that most cities and counties require permits. Check with yours.
- With public utility companies or delivery services, be **ALERT** to photo IDs, but not to rely solely on a uniform and credentials, especially if you did not make the arrangements. Call company to confirm, ask why you were not notified. Advise company of the questioned solicitors.
- **AVOID** letting strangers into your house.
- **AVOID** and never be distracted. Con artists work in teams and a partner may use the rear of the house to gain entry.

August 26

- If arriving home and you find your door or a window open and suspect someone inside, **AVOID** and "DON'T GO IN THE HOUSE."
- Leave immediately and call 9-1-1.
- DO NOT HANG UP, BUT STAY ON THE PHONE AND LISTEN TO THE DISPATCHER'S INSTRUCTIONS.
- Wait in a safe place and advise dispatcher your location and who is with you.

August 27

Be ALERT, AWARE And AVOID...

Labor Day is a holiday celebrated on the first Monday in September in the United States and Canada. Dedicated to the social and economic achievements of workers. It was first celebrated on Tuesday, September 5, 1882 and is also an unofficial end of summer.

- **AVOID.** Don't drink and drive.
- Be **AWARE** to use a sunscreen to block the damaging ultraviolet rays. Choose a sunscreen made for children with a sun protection factor (SPF) of at least 15. Apply 15 to 30 minutes before going out. Try to keep your child out of the sun when the peak ultraviolet rays occur, between 10 a.m. and 4 p.m. Be **ALERT** to dress your child in lightweight cotton clothing with long sleeves, long pants, and hat with wide brim. Use a beach umbrella or similar object to keep child in the shade as much as possible.

August 28

ARE YOU UNIQUE *TRIPLE A*™?

ALERT...

- What's in your trash? Do you shred bills, vital documents? Do you throw out boxes that display valuables (like a new 60" plasma HD TV box), prominently on the curb in front of your house, awaiting trash pickup? Or were you **ALERT** to carefully cut up the box before you discard in the trash bin, not outside of container?
- If leaving for a couple of days, a week, were you **ALERT** to cancel deliveries, such as newspapers, UPS, FEDEX, mail. Were you **ALERT** to have someone mow the lawn, take out the garbage, remove garbage cans, and discard throw-away papers?
- Be **ALERT** to use timers for water sprinklers, outdoor/indoor lights, appliances.

August 29

AWARE...

- Are vehicles that are usually in the driveway not there? Vehicles in the driveway not being used for days on end?
- Are you **AWARE** if a burglar has access to the home because of lack of security measures?
- Do you use the same schedules daily? Are you **AWARE** most residential burglaries take place during work hours, because often homes are unoccupied during these hours? When do you leave for work? When do you return from work? Do you come home for lunch?

August 30

- **AVOID** open blinds and curtains that can advertise items in home.
- Use exterior lighting and motion detectors to minimize burglar concealment.
- Have gardener continue outdoor work while on vacation.
- **AVOID** giving out "on vacation" and schedule in e-mails and phone messages.
- Notify police and neighbors upon your return.
- If you have to park your car outside overnight, **AVOID** leaving your garage door opener in your car to **AVOID** thieves gaining access to your home through the garage. Ensure that doors that lead to your house via the garage are locked securely and are hollow core doors.

August 31

KEY TO *THE UNIQUE TRIPLE A™*

Community crime prevention programs or strategies aim at changes in community infrastructure, culture, or the physical environment in order to decrease or lessen crime opportunities, such as burglary, gang violence, or neighborhood disarray. It involves citizens in shared efforts to be crime prevention pro-active with neighbors, community, law enforcement, and your city or county government. Participate in public forums, city council, or county supervisor meetings that allow residents to talk with elected and appointed leaders about crime and violence prevention needs. Get them involved in your community.

Together, communities can create a negative environment for crime. Remember, police and private patrol services are unable to be there 24-hours a day. Don't let them react after a crime. Be pro-active.

BONUS SAFETY TIP

Work together with neighbors to establish safe conditions in your neighborhood - a physical environment that doesn't invite crime or offer opportunities for violence to brew. With a group of neighbors, scan streets, yards, alleys, playgrounds, ball fields, parks, and other areas. Look with a child's eye; even invite some children to go with you. Ask your police department or sheriff's office if they'll provide pointers or other help. Look for things like overgrown lots, abandoned vehicles or appliances, public play areas blocked from public view, intersections and streets that need lighting or traffic control improvements, unsafe equipment or structures, abandoned buildings, hazards in nearby businesses or commercial areas, and signs of vandalism, especially graffiti.

Volunteer to build a stronger community. Volunteering profoundly impacts the people and communities serves. Nonprofit and civic organizations, Neighborhood Watch are win-win propositions for making a difference.

"Volunteering is the ultimate exercise in democracy. You vote in elections once a year, but when you volunteer, you vote every day about the kind of community you want to live in. Make a difference."

~ UNKNOWN

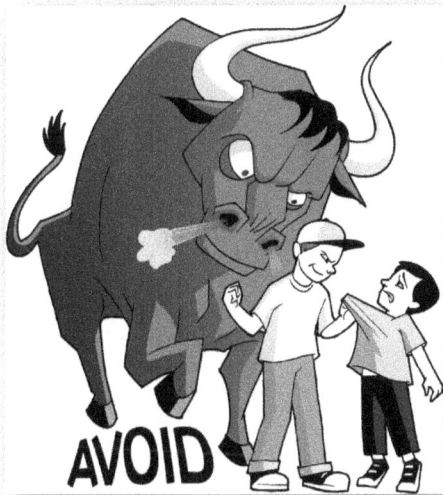

September

SCHOOL DAYS

———

Take The Bull(ying) By The Horns

September 1

FOR THE PARENTS

SCHOOL SMART

<u>Be School-Zone Smart...</u>

When it's back to school season, motorists should pay extra attention.

- Drive without distractions. **AVOID** using cell phone, eating, adjusting radio dials, or taking eyes away from the road while behind wheel.
- **AVOID** dropping off kids at a location where they have to cross the street.
- Be **ALERT** and **AWARE** around playgrounds and school zones where children may dart out into the street and from in-between parked cars.
- Obey school-zone speed limits.

September 2

WHAT IS BULLYING?

There are many definitions, but summarized, it is:

- The fighting, name-calling, teasing, threatening, or excluding someone repeatedly and over time.
- Unwanted, aggressive behavior among school-aged children that involves a real or perceived power imbalance, such as size or popularity.
- Physical, social, and emotional harm.
- Hurting another person to get something.

Bullying can affect the person being bullied in many ways:

- May lose sleep or feel sick.
- May want to skip school.
- May even be thinking about suicide.
- Feels hopeless, helpless.

September 3

- Teach children and teens to resolve problems without fighting.
- Talk to them about other ways they can work out problems such as walking away, talking it out, sticking with friends, or telling school staff. Explain that fighting leads to injury or earning a reputation as a bully.
- Be **ALERT** and **AWARE** of every concern they tell you, their emotions, feelings, and behaviors toward the incident.
- Be **ALERT** and look for warning signs/red flags, such as a sudden drop in grades, torn clothing, bruises, loss of friends, withdrawn, or refuses to go to school.
- Are your children happy in school? Talk to them about their day and if they saw anyone being bullied, or anything else that makes them feel uncomfortable.
- Remember and be **AWARE** that it may be difficult for young adults or teenagers to communicate. It may be due to peer pressure or they were involved.

September 4

- Keep an open dialogue. Decide on what to do together.
- Stay **AWARE** of their internet use, who they chat with, e-mail, and what sites they visit.
- Enroll them in extracurricular activities such as community programs, fun classes.
- Kids think they are cooler or smarter than their parents, and often embarrassed. Let them know if anything (or anyone, online social media) makes them uncomfortable, they can talk to you.
- Listen to what they say and take their concerns and worries seriously.
- Be **AWARE** you are listening, and not interrupting or giving opinions.
- Be **AWARE** that even if you know how to handle it and feel no big deal, this is a big deal to them.

September 5

- Sharpen your parenting skills.
- Emphasize and build on your children's strengths.
- Be **AWARE** to set clear rules about acceptable activities in advance.
- Work with other parents in your neighborhood to start a block-parent program.
- Put a high value on education and help your child do his best in school.
- Be **ALERT** to spend special time with each child and do everything possible to prevent them dropping out of school.
- Help your kids identify positive role models and heroes, especially people in your community.
- Be **AWARE** to praise them for doing well and encourage them to do their very best.

September 6

- It's important to discuss gangs and the problems they can create with your child.
- Tell them that you disapprove of gangs and don't want to see them hurt or arrested.
- Tell them that you see them as special and worth protecting to help them with any problems they might have.
- Tell them that family members don't keep secrets from each other and that it is important that you really want to be **ALERT, AWARE,** and listen to what they have to say.
- Make them feel good about themselves, their talents, skills, their contributions to society.

September 7

PARENTS AND OUTER SPACE ATTACKS

Cyberbullying happens when kids bully each other through electronic technology (cell phones, computers, tablets, social media sites, text messages, chat rooms, websites), with emails, mean text messages, rumors via e-mail or posted on social media sites, embarrassing photos, videos, or false profiles. Cyberbullying messages and images can be posted anonymously and distributed quickly to a very wide audience. It can be difficult and sometimes impossible to trace the source.

- Be **AWARE** of the sites your kids visit and their online activities.
- Have a sense of what they do online and in texts.
- Be **ALERT** you can install parental control filtering software or monitoring programs.
- Tell them that as a responsible parent you may review their online communications if you feel there is a concern.

September 8

PARENTS AND SCHOOL BULLYING

- Ask the school if students are monitored when they use the internet, or if there are blocking devices to prevent them access to explicit websites.
- Ask the school about their safety and emergency plans, and if students are **AWARE** of them.
- Is the school **ALERT** and **AWARE** of bullying issues and how are they handling them? Policies?
- Be **AWARE** and ask if there were any recent issues?
- How are local police, students, and parents involved in the school? And can be?
- What emergencies have been considered and planned for?

September 9

- Does the school implement visitor ID cards?
- Are there identification cards for faculty, staff, and/or students?
- What other security measures are in place for identifying students who do not attend the school?
- Be **AWARE** to ascertain what the policies are when students are involved in bullying and violence.
- Is there school security staff, and if so, are they in uniform or in plain clothes?
- Be **AWARE** and become involved in your child's school activities, PTA, field trips, and volunteer work, such as helping out in class or the lunchroom.
- **AVOID** being a bystander, be accountable and report immediately to school and law enforcement any bullying incidents.

September 10

PARENTS: BULLYING AND DAUGHTERS

- The 2004 movie, *Mean Girls,* depicts cliques, queen bees, and wannabes as a satire comedy; however, the experiences are real. Rent it and get your child's feedback.
- Typically, "mean girls" are not always big, tough-looking. They can be popular, do well in school, and don't get into fights. Instead they spread gossip, rumors, excludes others, shares secrets, and tease other girls about their athletic ability, hair, intelligence, looks, race, height, or weight. Most likely you will find them bullying in a group, bullying others to join in, or use pressure to get involved.
- Is your child one of the "mean girls"? Remember, and be **AWARE** that it may be difficult for young girls or teenagers to communicate to a parent or adult. Make them feel at ease.

September 11

- If your daughter is involved, in order to move forward, forgive. Sometimes a bully may be coming from a broken place, parents not spending enough time with them, both parents working or arguing, a single-parent household, and at times, no family time at dinnertime.
- Reach out and set aside a quiet time to talk and listen regarding their concerns.
- Arrange a "lady-fun" day devoted to them and get involved with them.
- Be **AWARE** to be a good example. Don't gossip or make fun of others in front of young girls.
- Talk to them about their friends, what they do together, and how they treat each other. Ask them what makes a good friend, and whether their friends have these qualities.

September 12

PARENTS: BULLYING AND SONS

Steps for Parents and Sons...

- Accusations can't be taken lightly.
- Be **ALERT** first to talk with your son about his perspective on what is happening and why he might be engaging in it.
- Is it to get attention, be one of the popular school boys, to be accepted or forced, to **AVOID** being a victim, a lack of meaningful friendships, entitlement or contempt, or to gain some kind of special power or favor?
- As with any gender, start by taking a look at what goes on at home. Is there a father or male adult in the house who is not a role model?

September 13

- Be **ALERT** to think before going on the offensive.
- Teach him to learn more effective problem-solving and relationship-building skills.
- Consider ways to respond to the good intentions that might underlie the words or actions you find offensive.
- Be **AWARE** if there is someone else he can trust about his issues, concerns?
- Build networks of social support, involving other kids as well as adults.
- Help him act with self-confidence.
- Involve him in activities outside of school. This way he can make friends in a different social circle.

NOTE:

National Grandparents Day is celebrated annually on the first Sunday after Labor Day.

September 14

Children who feel good about themselves and are proud of their achievements are less likely to **AVOID** and participate in bullying activities, so you can also help your children by emphasizing community, empathy, friendship-building, and respect.

- Build a family climate of mutual respect.
- Ask a teacher or a school counselor if your child is facing any problems at school, struggling with a particular subject, or has difficulty making friends. Ask them for advice on how you and your child can work through the problem.
- Be **ALERT** and **AWARE**. Ask yourself if someone at home is bullying your child. Kids who bully are often bullied themselves by a parent or family member.

<u>NOTES</u>:

September 15

TEEN STRESS

The American Psychological Association says adolescents report higher stress levels during the school year, mostly from extracurricular rosters, social demands, and typical teenage drama. Long-term chronic stress can affect teens cognitively, making focusing on schoolwork difficult, increasing risk for depression, anxiety, and vulnerability to bullying.

So How Can You Help…

Look for changes in behavior, such as:

- Are they less happy than usual? More irritable?
- Are they bailing out of social activities, texting less, gaining weight, or complaining about headaches?
- Eating well? Serve healthy snacks and schedule family meals when possible, which will also promote communication. Add laughter, like a movie or a family pizza night.

September 16

Bullying vs Violence. There is a fine line in the differences. Violence may be defined as doing harm to another, whether physical or mental. Bullying could be considered a form of violence, but differs, because it usually occurs when one person or group of people singles out another person with the intent of being mean through name-calling, threating, spreading rumors, hitting or social exclusion.

Bullying behavior is generally repeated over a period of time until it becomes a pattern and victims feel helpless, unable to fight back, or defend themselves.

Though violence is generally seen as an unacceptable type of behavior, more people accept bullying as a normal part of life.

While violence and violent crimes have generally been decreasing, bullying has not.

Violence is against the law, while bullying generally isn't unless it crosses the line into harassment or assault.

September 17

FOR THE STUDENT

- Settle arguments with words, not fists or weapons.
- If you don't know how, learn how.
- Be **AWARE** and report crimes or suspicious activities to the police, school authorities.
- Tell a school official immediately if you are **AWARE** or see another student with a gun, knife, or other weapon.
- Tell a teacher, parent, or trusted adult if you are worried about a bully, threats, or violence by another student.
- Stay **ALERT** walking and coming home from school.
- Be **AWARE** and keep your focus on your surroundings.
- Walk purposely, stand tall, and make eye contact with people around you.

September 18

- Learn safe routes for traveling to and from school, and stick to them.
- Be **ALERT** and know where, or who to go to, seek help.
- Stay **ALERT, AWARE,** and know where you're going and the safest way to get there, particularly when moving about the city during hours of darkness.
- Walk/run in well-lit areas avoiding short cuts through alleys and parking lots.
- Get involved in your school's anti-violence activities.
- **AVOID** being pressured to join gangs.
- **AVOID** places and people associated with them.

September 19

CAMPUS AND PERSONAL SAFETY

- Stay **AWARE** and **AVOID** walking around campus alone at night.
- Use the buddy system, walk in groups to and from campus buildings and parking lots.
- Does your campus have police escort services?
- If you see someone being victimized immediately call campus police.
- Stay on well-lit, regular traveled walks or pathways.
- **AVOID** thick shrubbery, bushes, alleyways, or any other areas where an assailant is lurking or hiding.
- **AVOID** secluded or dimly-lit areas. Report lights that are out and any hazardous conditions immediately to campus authorities.
- If you need transportation during evening hours, check if your school offers walking escorts or mobile transport scheduled services.

September 20

- If you think you are being followed, cross the street, and if necessary, keep crossing back and forth, yell, scream, and move toward a public, well-lit area, a campus building, business, pull a fire alarm, or anything to attract attention to summon assistance.
- Be **AWARE** of locations of emergency phones and fire extinguishers in all campus buildings and your hallways.
- Ascertain a map of campus, emergency phones, and extinguisher locations. Be **ALERT** where they are located.
- Report suspicious activities and/or persons immediately.
- What are the campus safety policies for students who have classes in the evenings or use the library in the evening? Check security or escort services.
- Always be **ALERT** and **AWARE** of what is going on around you.
- List locations of outside campus phones below.

September 21

Athletic Facilities...

- **AVOID** using athletic facilities alone, especially after dark or during off-hours.
- Use the buddy system, work out with a friend, and make arrangements to leave the gym together.
- Confine running and jogging to the daylight hours and to open, well-traveled areas.
- **AVOID** bringing personal items of value to the gym.
- **AVOID** leaving your keys unattended anywhere.
- Use a lock on your gym locker.
- **AVOID** showering alone, especially evening hours.

September 22

Bicycles, Motorbikes...

- Keep them securely chained and locked when not in use.
- **AVOID** parking or storing in dimly-lit areas.
- Engrave or permanently mark an identifying number, record that number and bike information with school police, and keep a copy for your files.
- Park in a well-lit location, or by a nearby security camera.
- Chain and lock to a secure unmovable item when leaving it unattended.
- Besides alarms, cables, and chains, be **AWARE** of new anti-theft products, such as the disc lock mounted onto a brake disc. A locking pin goes through either a cutaway space inside disc or one of its holes to prevent wheel from turning.

September 23

- Some alarms incorporate a current drain sensor that monitors the electrical system to detect when someone is trying to hot wire a motorcycle.

- Be **AWARE** that more expensive systems send a text message to your phone if tampered with, even if you're unable to hear the alarm.

- Motorcycle covers can disguise and make motorcycles less likely to be targeted. Purchase one you can place a lock on to prevent removal.

- Check with your motorcycle insurance company if they offer a discount for anti-theft devices installed on your motorcycle.

- When selecting a locking device, be **AWARE** that some come in bright colors to help serve as a visual deterrent.

- Be **AWARE** you have the right insurance protection for your motorcycle, if stolen.

September 24

<u>Corridors, Elevators/Hallways, Restrooms, Stairs...</u>

- While waiting for a campus elevator alone, **AVOID** getting in with people who look out of place, or behave in a strange or threatening manner. **AVOID** going in. Wait for its return without the stranger.
- In an elevator, immediately stand or stay close to the control panel, where you have access to the alarm and floor buttons.
- If you find yourself in an elevator with someone who makes you nervous, get off as soon as possible.
- **AVOID** trouble spots, such as out-of-the way stairwells and corridors.
- **AVOID** poorly lighted areas.
- Be cautious when using restrooms. **AVOID** restrooms that are isolated or poorly lighted.
- **AVOID** using all of the above alone.

September 25

Dorms...

- Keep the doors to your room and windows locked at all times.
- **AVOID** putting your personal address on school books, binders.
- **AVOID** keeping your room, residence, and vehicle keys on the same ring.
- If you lose your keys to your residence or room, have the locks changed.
- On campus, residents should notify campus authorities immediately.
- **AVOID** keeping large amounts of cash in your room.

September 26

- If you receive obscene or harassing telephone calls, or calls with no one on the other end, HANG UP and immediately notify campus police and roommate.
- Report suspicious persons or activities in your residence hall.
- **AVOID** propping open exterior doors to residence halls.
- **AVOID** allowing unescorted visitors into the hall.

September 27

Driving And Parking...

- If you are driving back to campus and think you are being followed, keep out of isolated areas, sound your horn, turn on emergency lights, drive toward campus police building, or busy streets, open stores, shopping centers, or 24-hour emergency facilities such as hospitals, fire, police, gas stations.

- **AVOID** returning to campus until you have sought help.

- When parking at night, choose well-lit areas.

- Be **ALERT** and **AWARE** of surroundings.

- Before, during, and after exiting, stay **ALERT** and **AWARE** to your surroundings, people, and shadows.

- Keep keys between fingers as a defense weapon.

- If possible, call security for an escort and wait in car. Be **ALERT** your key fob has a panic alarm button. Use if you are near your car.

September 28

Personal Property...

- **AVOID** allowing your property or valuables to be unattended at any time.
- Make a list of your valuables, electronics, including make, model, and serial number.
- Permanently mark your personal property and valuables with electronic engravers.
- If you find your room has been entered, **AVOID** going in, and call campus police immediately.
- **AVOID** leaving books, handbags, or valuables unattended in any school facilities or locations.
- **AVOID** giving student locker combinations to anyone.
- Mark your books with your name or some type of markings for easy identification should they get stolen.
- If your books, handbag, or other property are stolen, notify school authorities immediately

September 29

DON'T INVITE TROUBLE

- **AVOID** wearing expensive clothing and jewelry. Keep purses and wallets close to your body.
- Use ATMS during the day and have all deposit slips prepared prior to going to ATM.
- **AVOID** wearing clothing or footwear that restricts your movement.
- **AVOID** jogging during evening or late hours.
- Doing your part means being **AWARE** of your vulnerability and following the suggestions outlined.
- It means being **ALERT** for suspicious or criminal activity and conditions that may represent a potential danger or threat to you.
- It means **AVOIDING** suspicious places, people, and reporting crimes.
- Unreported crimes cannot be solved. Without reports, you allow the perpetrators to commit additional and more serious crimes.

September 30

GET INTO THE ACT

Here are some suggestions/ideas to get involved.

- Parents can take an active role in formulating the safety and security plans at their children's school.
- Parents can help develop recreational and educational programs for young people so that they will have better alternatives than drugs, alcohol, and gangs, and can benefit from adult supervision and mentoring.
- Young people can start a conflict resolution program at school.
- Young people can report incidents of discrimination or hate crime to parents and teachers.

Bullying in any form is done because when the bully can make someone feel bad or hurt, the bully gains power over that person. Power makes them feel like they are better than another person, makes them feel good about themselves, and makes them stand out and gain attention from other kids and adults.

AVOID letting anyone take away your power, self-esteem, and confidence. Be confident.

BONUS SAFETY TIP

<u>Were You AWARE?</u>...

The word "bully" used to mean the total opposite of what it means now? Five-hundred years ago, it meant *friend, family member,* or *sweetheart.*

The root of the word comes from the Dutch *boel,* meaning *lover* or *brother.* Big change!

Watching the bully is a way to bully "vicariously" and the same as being the bully. The "watchers" feel they are getting their frustrations out by hurting someone even though they are not doing the hurting.

- They are entertained by the bullying.
- They want to side with the bully because to do so makes they feel strong and powerful. Siding with the victim would make them weak.

Risk reduction is like self-esteem.
It doesn't need anyone's permission but yours.

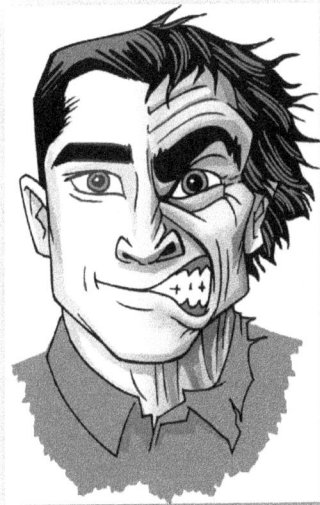

October

BOO!

———

Trick or Treat Horrors Of Domestic Violence

October 1

WHAT IS DOMESTIC VIOLENCE/ABUSE?

First of all, it is a crime by law. In summary, domestic violence is defined as abuse, emotional or physical, enacted by one or both partners involved in a relationship. It is a pattern of abusive and/or harassing behavior, actions, verbal threats by a partner, to gain or maintain power and control over another intimate partner.

Domestic violence can include physical, sexual, emotional, economic, psychological actions or threats of actions and behaviors, to exert control to blame, coerce, frighten, humiliate, hurt, injure, intimidate, isolate, manipulate, terrorize, threaten, or wound the partner (also includes breaking into victim's home, destroy or steal victim's property). Abuse can occur between married, cohabiting, dating, heterosexual, homosexual, regardless of socioeconomic status, race, religion, or education levels of those involved.

Domestic violence is a repetitive pattern in people's lives. Victims or witnesses in childhood are likely to be abusers.

October 2

- Domestic violence is everyone's responsibility. It is a social and moral responsibility and always bad for children.

- Are you **AWARE** that violence erodes communities by reducing productivity, decreasing property values?

- Be **AWARE** that domestic violence is more than just a family problem. It is a crime enacted by any person against any age to threaten, physically and/or sexually assault, beat, emotionally abuse, or otherwise harm another person, even if they are married.

- From infants to the elderly, it affects people in all stages of life.

- Abuse is also common in teens who are dating. It often happens through controlling behaviors, jealousy, and possessiveness. The abuser uses fear and threats to gain power and control over the other person.

- Power and control include coercion threats, intimidation, economic, emotional, physical abuse, isolation, using children, and blaming.

Source: National Coalition Against Domestic Violence at http//www.ncadv.org

October 3

Did You Know?...

- An estimated 1.3 million women are victims of physical assault by an intimate partner each year.
- Be **AWARE** that 1 in 3 women and 1 in 4 men have been victims of some form of physical violence by an intimate partner within their lifetime.
- 30 to 60 percent of perpetrators of intimate partner violence also abuse children in the household.
- Domestic violence is one of the most chronically, underreported crimes.
- Approximately 20 percent of the 1.5 million people who experience intimate partner violence annually obtain protection orders.
- 1 of every 2 families in the United States is involved in domestic violence at some time.

Source: National Coalition Against Domestic Violence at http//www.ncadv.org

October 4

Did You Know?...

- Domestic violence and child abuse often occur in the same family and are linked to consequences for all family members and the community.

- Children exposed to domestic violence are at greater risk for substance abuse, juvenile pregnancy, and criminal behavior than those raised in homes without violence.

- Studies have shown that children from violent homes exhibit signs of more aggressive behavior, such as bullying, and more likely to be involved in fighting and aggressive abuse to others as well as animals. Many, including children, survive violence and are left with permanent physical and emotional scars.

- Prevention and early intervention efforts can be effective in reducing domestic violence and child abuse behavior.

Source: National Coalition Against Domestic Violence at http://www.ncadv.org

October 5

In 1984, October was designated as Crime Prevention Month through a presidential proclamation. Local and national law enforcement agencies, battered women's advocates, organizations, and family services, such as National Coalition Against Domestic Violence (NCADV), designated October as National Domestic Violence Awareness Month. It is a good time to renew community and neighborhood commitment to raising **AWARENESS** and preventing this serious crime.

The Unique Triple A™ is one resource that can aid in preventative measures to be **AWARE, ALERT,** and to **AVOID** and diffuse violent situations, or get away.

October 6

<u>**A Profile of Victims...**</u>

- Low self-esteem, lacks clear self-identity.
- Socially unsophisticated and shy.
- Accepts responsibility for batterer's behavior.
- Uses sex to establish intimacy.
- Believes no one can help, and they must be self-sufficient.
- Reserved, passive, and become withdrawn under stress.
- Strong belief in traditional gender roles within the family.
- Feels guilty, but denies terror and anger.

October 7

A Profile Of Batterers...

- Low self-esteem.
- Alternates between violence and being regretful.
- Blames others for their behavior.
- Socially isolated.
- Becomes paranoid under stress.
- Does not believe the violent behavior should have negative consequences.
- Has severe stress reactions, with which they cope by drinking and battering.
- Uses sex as an act of aggression, often to bolster self-esteem.
- Strong belief in traditional gender roles within the family.
- Pathologically jealous.

October 8

Sometimes after experiencing a traumatic domestic event, strong emotions, jitters, sadness, guilt, depression may all be part of this normal reaction.

Nightmares, headaches, back pains, smoking, or use of alcohol or drugs, anger, tension, fear are some of the common reactions.

Abuse can occur through the use of electronic technology, such as cell phones, computers, tablets, social media sites, text messages, chat, websites that includes e-mails, rumors, embarrassing pictures, videos, or fake profiles.

Are you **AWARE** of your reactions to abuse? List some below and in a journal.

October 9

THE DOMESTIC VIOLENCE CYCLE

The behavior of abusers don't always start with physical abuse. Physical abuse is only one part of a system of abusive behaviors the abuser uses to get and keep control over another person, and/or family.

Please be **AWARE** of the cycles of domestic violence and which stage you are in. Consider this if you decide to let the abuser know you are leaving. Consider how (in-person, tele-phone, or other type notification), and when to leave safely.

Tension-Building...

• Criticizes, angry gestures, threats, coercions.

Violence...

• Physical and sexual attacks, threats.

Seduction/Honeymoon...

• Apologies, blaming, promises to change, gifts.

October 10

Abuser may not display every behavior in each cycle, and not necessarily in the order listed; however, use caution if even one or two behaviors are displayed. Start planning for your safety.

Uses Intimidation or Fear...

- Has not struck you, but angers quickly or shows aggressive behavior.
- Intimidates, jealous, possessive, you feel afraid or unsafe.
- Uses looks, actions, gestures.
- May smash things, destroy or hide your property.
- May abuse pets.
- May display a weapon.

Male Privilege/Entitlement...

- King of the castle.
- Makes all the decisions.
- Defines men and women's roles.
- Treats you like a servant.

October 11

Coercion and Threats...

- Makes and/or carries out threats to do something to hurt you.
- Threatens to leave or commit suicide.
- If arrested or police called, makes you drop the charges.
- May engage you in illegal things.

Emotional Abuse...

- Puts you down and/or makes you feel bad about yourself.
- Plays mind games.
- Makes you think you are crazy.
- Humiliates.
- Makes you feel guilty. It's all your fault.
- You made him do it.

October 12

Uses Economic Abuse...

- Prevents or keeps you from a job, or from being independent.
- Gives you an allowance, or makes you beg or ask for money.
- Takes or controls your money.
- Does not let, or allow you to know about, or have access to, family income or bank account.

Uses Isolation...

- Controls what you do, who you see, talk to, where you go, buy, or even read.
- Limits or controls outside involvement.
- Uses jealousy to justify actions.
- May stalk you or show up unexpectedly wherever you are.

October 13

Blames, Denies...

- Makes light of the abuse.
- Not take your concerns about the abuse seriously.
- Denies the abuse.
- Shifts the responsibility for abusive behavior.
- Says you caused it.

Uses Children...

- Makes you feel guilty about the children.
- Threatens to take children away.
- Uses children to relay messages.

October 14

<u>**Help for Abused and Battered Women...**</u>

You are not alone. There are people waiting to help, and resources such as **<u>restraining orders, domestic violence helplines, shelters, legal aid,</u>** and **<u>advocates</u>**. Please refer to a few resources listed under Resources. However, always check and contact your local community for immediate help for resources and shelters.

Be **AWARE** if you are in danger and call 9-1-1.

- You are not to blame for being battered or mistreated.
- You are not the cause of your partner's abusive behavior.
- You deserve to be treated with respect.
- You and your children deserve a safe and happy life.
- You deserve to live free from fear.
- You are not alone. People are waiting to help.

October 15

TEMPORARY RESTRAINING ORDER (TRO)

Simply put, a TRO, or order of protection, are injunctions issued by a judge intended to protect, by law, those who fear for their own and/or children's safety. They prohibit the abuser from any contact or communication (in person, by phone, at residence, work, or other location), or actions that are likely to cause harm.

A restraining order can be granted immediately, without a hearing and without any notice to the opposing party. Temporary Restraining Orders are intended to last only until a hearing can take place. If a restraining order is violated, the abused should call 9-1-1 and report the situation. The violating party can be arrested immediately and taken into custody. In some states, the police can give the victim a short term Emergency Protection Order (EPO), when the abuser is arrested, which gives victim time to obtain a longer term order.

October 16

Be **AWARE** that the police can enforce a restraining order and arrest the abuser when abuser violates it and the conditions set by the judge. Orders can include many different provisions, depending on each case, including:

Move Out Provision: Requiring the abuser to move out of a home shared with the victim.

Stay Away Provision: Ordering the abuser to stay at least a certain number of yards or feet away from the victim, the home, job, school, and car. The stay-away distance can vary by state, judge, or the lethality of the situation, but is often at least 100 yards or 300 feet.

Obtain a protection order by filing with your local superior court. Be **AWARE** to follow your state law to present evidence. The police can sometimes serve the papers to the abuser for you. A copy of your TRO must always be in your possession and on file with the police departments where you live and work.

October 17

Be **ALERT** to let your employer, neighbors, close friends, and family know about the restraining order. Ask that they contact the police if they see the other party near you. If a restraining order is violated, call the police immediately.

Protect your children by notifying school administration, teachers, childcare centers, babysitters, and neighbors of the restraining order and requesting that they contact police if they suspect the order is being violated.

You should also keep a cell phone on you at all times and be ready to call 9-1-1 if you spot your former abuser.

October 18

HOTLINES, LEGAL AID, SHELTERS

If you think you are a victim of domestic violence, please seek help in your local community or at the summarized resources listed at the back of the book under RESOURCES.

Your local community resources can answer questions and assist with vital information from housing, separation, how to obtain a TRO, guidelines, help in filling forms, shelters, and additional information.

A shelter is a refuge center for battered victims and their children, and kept confidential from abuser. The shelter provides basic living needs such as food, childcare, counseling, support groups, employment, and educational and health-related programs. The length of time stayed is limited, but most shelters will also help find a permanent home, job, and other things needed to start a new life.

October 19

SAFETY WHILE AT HOME

- You must be **AWARE** to do safety planning for yourself and your family at home and at work.
- Be **AWARE** there are things you can do that may be helpful in planning for your safety while still at home and for your future safety.
- Make a safety plan. Call a domestic violence hotline or victim advocacy, or call your local police agency for assistance.
- Teach children emergency escape actions and proper telephone use.
- Practice an escape plan for emergencies, and go over it with a counselor, domestic violence prevention officer, or victim advocate.
- Do not share this safety plan with anyone who may reveal your plans to the abuser.

October 20

- Choose a code word that you can use with friends, neighbors, family, and children to **ALERT** them to call for help.
- Ask neighbors to listen, watch, and call for police assistance if they see suspicious people, activities, or hear arguing from your home.
- When violence seems imminent, **AVOID** the kitchen (knives), bathroom, and rooms that do not have exits to the outside.
- Notify someone immediately if you think that your abuser is about to become violent. Use noisemakers such as a whistle or personal alarm to summon assistance.
- Be **AWARE** you can use a deactivated cell phone to call 9-1-1 for emergencies free of charge.
- Always keep change for a pay phone set-aside in a safe place if you escape outside without a cell phone or unable to reach neighbors.

October 21

- Be **ALERT** and take care of yourself.
- Eat healthy, well-balanced meals and drink plenty of water. **AVOID** drugs and alcohol.
- They may seem to help with the stress, but in the long run, they create additional problems and increase the stress you are already feeling.
- Get plenty of sleep. Exercise on a regular basis.
- Increase your independence by opening a bank account, getting credit cards in your own name, and obtaining job skills.
- Talk to a counselor, social worker, law enforcement. Seek help.
- Keep a journal of incidents, your feelings, reactions in a safe and secure place.
- A list with dates/times of violent incidents and/or abuse could aid in obtaining a restraining or protective order.

October 22

Getting Out And Preparing To Leave...

- Be **ALERT** and **AWARE** that the danger may get worse while attempting to escape or after leaving a violent relationship.
- Talk to your local law enforcement or a domestic violence advocate about obtaining restraining orders or an order of protection (see RESOURCES).
- Revisit the safety plan with them.
- List vital contact resources, numbers below.

October 23

MAKE AN ESCAPE BAG

- Prepare a bag, box, or suitcase filled with things you will need WHEN you leave.
- Keep it in a safe place away from home, if possible.
- **AVOID** taking items that may **ALERT** the abuser to your plan.
- Other than law enforcement and domestic violence advocates, **AVOID** telling anyone about the bag or plans to leave.
- Obtain the 1991 movie, *Sleeping with the Enemy*. There are some lessons to learn.

October 24

The Escape Bag...

Should contain: a change of clothing, spare keys to house and car, medication needed, your journal and any photos of injuries, copy of your restraining or order of protection, address book/phone numbers, photo of abuser for ID purposes, identification (birth certificates, driver's license, green cards, work permits, and/or social security cards for you and the children), personal hygiene and toiletry products, divorce, custody or injunction papers, diapers, formula, toys (if applicable), blankets, emergency numbers, copies of car, health and life insurance documents, cash, credit cards, bank books (Did you open a separate bank account?).

NOTES:

October 25

Protecting Yourself After You Leave...

Keeping yourself safe from your abuser is just as important after you've left as before. To protect yourself, you may need to relocate so your former partner can't find you. If you have children, they may need to switch schools.

- If you feel unsafe, **AVOID** being left alone. Have a relative/friend with you, when possible. Be **ALERT** to make sure your relatives/friends are **AWARE** of your breakup.
- Be **AWARE** of your surroundings and who is watching/stalking you.
- Pay attention to your ex-partner's reaction to the breakup.
- Calling 9-1-1 and filing a restraining order should always be considered for your safety.

"We have to let go of all blame, all attacking, all judging, to free our inner selves to attract what we say we want."

~ JOE VITALE, Author, Life Coach

October 26

- Consider having your telephone numbers and new address unlisted, use a P.O. Box, or place in another person's name.

- Consider changing phone numbers (purchase a "burner phone"), e-mail, and if possible, moving out of town, city, or state.

- Be **AWARE** if your state offers a confidentiality program. It's a service that confidentially forwards your mail to your home. Keep your new location a secret.

- Cancel your old bank accounts and credit cards, especially if you shared them with your abuser. When you open new accounts, be sure to use a different bank.

- If you remain in the same area, be **ALERT** to change up your routine. Take a new route to work, **AVOID** places where your abuser might think to locate you, change any appointments he knows about, find new places to shop, run errands, or even change doctor, dentist.

- What about schools children attend? **ALERT** them about restraining orders against abuser.

October 27

SAFETY AT WORK

- Ask someone to screen your calls for awhile.
- Obtain a restraining or protection order and keep a copy with you.
- Plan an escape route (**AVOID** going to your car).
- Provide security or reception areas with a photo of the abuser.
- Request that your office or desk be placed in a safer location.
- Plan your entry and exit each day with different hours, routes.
- Request help from an employee assistance program.

October 28

CHILDREN

Because of their level of development, children and minors may not be able to know how to cope well with stress from a traumatic domestic violent event.

- It is natural for children to worry when stressful events occur in their lives.
- Talk to them about the issues and monitor them.
- Educators and professionals can help take steps to provide stability, support, and put the event into a more balanced context with information that can help them feel better.

October 29

THE CYCLE OF ABUSE

<u>Why Doesn't The Victim Leave?...</u>

It's the question many people ask when they learn that someone is being battered and abused. Getting out of an abusive relationship is not easy. The victim may think abuser will change, or afraid of what abuser will do if the abuser discovers victim is trying to leave. The "honeymoon cycle" or make-up cycle gives the victim a sense of love and hope it will all work out as the abuser promises it will never happen again.

It's even harder when the victim has been isolated from family and friends, financially and psychologically abused. They feel trapped, frightened, uncertain, and helpless.

Be **ALERT** and **AWARE** that help and resources are available, some even free. There are crisis hotlines, childcare, legal services, and job training to help with your needs.

October 30

MOST FREQUENTLY ASKED QUESTIONS

Can You Take Your Children With You When You Leave?...

Yes, if you can do so safely. The lives and safety of you and your children are a priority. Be **AWARE** you have the right to contact your local police agency and request them to stand by while you leave, whether the abuser is at the house or not. Make a police report with them for the abuse and he can be immediately arrested.

- Get legal advice regarding legal custody of children.

Where Do You Go?

- Please be **AWARE** of the shelters in your areas where staff can help you get legal and financial help, counseling, emotional support for you and your children.

October 31

THE HORRORS OF DOMESTIC VIOLENCE

"...he went completely crazy when he burned his hand. I thought he was going to put me through a window. He then punched a hole in a wall, threatened to kill me while our two children hid terrified... It was the second time he lost his temper that I realized he was 2 different people..."

"...sitting on the couch and out of nowhere felt a blow to the back of my head. My head was hurting...He pushed my head into the pillow and raped me..."

In 2000, emergency hospitals nationwide reported more than 2.5 million injuries were due to domestic violence. Americans suffered $2.2 million in medically related injuries. Total lifetime cost was $37 billion ($4 billion for medical treatment, $44 billion for lost productivity). Nearly 17,000 resulted in homicides costing society $22 billion in medical costs and lost productivity. Commonly used weapons: hands, belts, baseball bats, kitchen utensils, teeth. Physical and psychological abuse are linked to adverse effects including arthritis, chronic neck or back pain. Domestic violence is everyone's responsibility. It erodes communities by reducing productivity, decreasing property values.

A violent crime occurs every **26 SECONDS**
1 IN 3 Women experience domestic abuse from partners
1 IN 5 Women are survivors of rape

Source: 2007 American Journal of Preventative Medicine, Vol. 32, No. 6. http://www.cdc.gov/violenceprevention/pdf/medical_costs.pdf
Source: htttp://www.nomore.org.fbi.gov

BONUS SAFETY TIP

Abuse is never a one-time event with an abuser. The scars of domestic violence run deep and you may struggle with emotions, memories, or a sense of being in danger. The traumas can stay long after you've escaped the abusive situation. Counseling, therapy, and support groups can help you process what you've been through, speed recovery from emotional, physical, and psychological distress, learn how to build new and healthy relationships, move on, heal, and feel safe again.

To **AVOID** another abusive relationship, be **ALERT** and not so eager to jump into a new relationship. Be **AWARE** and wise to go slow, take the time to become a new you, and to understand how you got into the previous abusive relationship. Without taking the time to heal and learn, you risk falling back into abusive patterns with abusive partners.

"You are
Braver
than you believe,
Stronger
than you seem,
Smarter
than you think
&
Loved
more than you know."

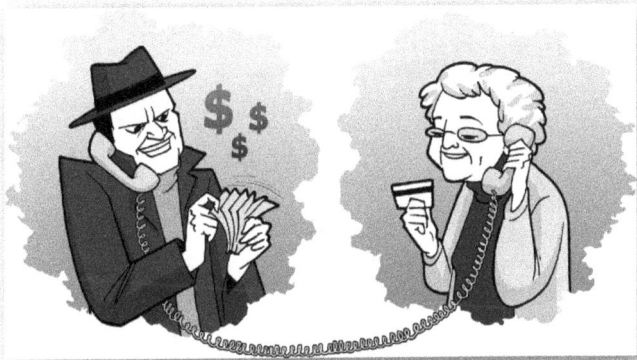

November

BOUNTY OF THANKS

———

Seniors Rule

November 1

With a large percentage of citizens over the age of 65 nation-wide, they are targets for a wide variety of crimes.

- Senior citizens currently represent the most rapidly growing segment of the population in the United States.
- As of latest available year data, 2009: one in every eight Americans is 65 or older which is 39.6 million people, or 12.9 percent of the US population.
- By year 2030, as "baby boomers" age and life expectancy increases, number will increase to estimated 72.1 million, twice number of 2000.
- In 2050, the number of Americans aged 65 and older is projected to be 88.5 million, more than double its projected population of 40.2 million in 2010.

Sources: U.S. Census Bureau. htpp://www.census.gov Senior Americans for Senior Citizens Month. **Detail:** Census Bureau Facts for Features: Older Americans Month: May 2010. htpp://www.fbi.gov

November 2

- Projected 2009 midyear world population, 65 and older, is 520 million.
- Projections indicate the number will increase to 1.53 billion by 2050.
- The percentage of the world's population, 65 and older, will increase from less than 8 percent to 17 percent over the period. By 2050, Europe's rate will be 29 percent.
- Number of countries with 20 percent or more of their population 65 and older in 2009 includes Germany, Italy, Japan, and Monaco.

NOTE:

Be **ALERT** Daylight Saving Time ends 2:00 a.m. the first Sunday in November, annually. Adjust clocks one hour to fall back.

Don't forget to change carbon monoxide and smoke alarm batteries.

Sources: International Data Base: http://www.census.gov/ipc htpp://www/idb/groups.php
Population Estimates: http://www.census.gov

November 3

Phone scams are on the rise! AVOID scams, such as the grandparent, "please don't tell my parents," or "get me out of jail," jury duty warrants, pigeon drop, bank examiner, telemarketing, police/fire/utility impersonators. Be **ALERT** and **AWARE** to question the legitimacy of the vow of secrecy and sense of urgency calls, send money scams.

The use of Green Dot cards (noted for the green dot image on card) is a relatively new wrinkle. In the past, scammers would have you wire money using Western Union or a similar service. Green Dot cards (prepaid MasterCard or Visa debit card where money is loaded onto the card for purchases or to pay bills) are a more sophisticated and efficient way for con artists to steal your cash.

Never act immediately no matter how dramatic the story may be. Verify the caller's identity by asking questions a stranger couldn't answer. Check things out with another family member even if you've been sworn to secrecy. Never wire money or load cash onto a debit card. **AVOID** giving out personal information, such as social security, bank PIN numbers, and passwords.

November 4

WHY SENIORS ARE TARGETED

The Unique Triple A™ goal is to have seniors learn to be **AWARE** and **ALERT** to potential elder crimes, and show them how to **AVOID** being victimized by scams and identity theft.

- Often have a retirement "nest egg," in their own home and/or have excellent credit, both of which are attractive features to the con person.

- Less likely or **AVOIDS** to report a fraud because they don't know who to report it to, are too ashamed of having been scammed, or do not know they have been scammed.

- When a senior victim does report a crime and there is an arrest, they often make poor witnesses.

- The effects of age on memory often make it difficult for them to serve as a good witness.

- Con artists can usually obtain the willing cooperation of the victim to complete the scheme.

- Scams work because the imposters play on seniors' fears and use a sense of urgency for them to weaken.

November 5

Be **ALERT** that the con artist ultimately will exploit his/her victim's assets including: life insurance benefits, pensions or annuities, "nest eggs," home equity, or other tangible property.

- **AVOID** being pressured into a verbal agreement or signing a contract.
- **AVOID** paying for products or services in advance.
- Get estimates and ask for references on home repair offers and other services.
- Be **AWARE** of unsolicited offers to make repairs to your home.
- **AVOID** the "tar roof" repair scheme from solicitors.

November 6

PROTECT YOUR INCOME

- Be **AWARE** and suspicious of anyone who offers you a chance for quick and easy wealth.
- If you are offered a deal that sounds too good to be true, it usually is.
- Be **ALERT** and wary of exaggerated claims for health and medical products, such as cures for cancer, arthritis, hair restorers, quick weight loss.
- Before buying any cure-alls, check with your doctor, pharmacist, or clinic.
- **AVOID** giving any details about your credit cards to phone solicitors, even if they offer you gifts, a free vacation, or a sweepstakes prize.
- Check out any "work-at-home" schemes with your local or state consumer protection agency.

"If something seems to be too good to be true, it's probably too good to be true."

November 7

- Understand completely what you are getting into.
- If you are not totally confident in the transaction, **DON'T SIGN ANYTHING!**
- Be **ALERT** and take the greatest care when signing any loan contracts.
- **AVOID** entering into an insurance or medical program without first verifying its authenticity.
- Use resources such as Better Business Bureau.
- Be **ALERT** and **AWARE** to always wait and talk it over with a trusted attorney, or legal aid, to consult first before getting into any contracts.
- Bottom line, NEVER trust anyone who calls or shows up at your door, demands money.
- **AVOID** GIVING OUT PERSONAL INFORMATION OF ANY KIND.

"People are always asking me when I'm going to retire. Why should I? I've got it two ways— I'm still making movies, and I'm a senior citizen, so I can see myself at half price."

~ GEORGE BURNS

November 8

BANK SCAMS

Never withdraw money from your bank accounts for anyone except YOURSELF.

- Be **AWARE** of scams, such as pigeon drops and bank examiners (see GLOSSARY).
- **AVOID** and walk away from solicitations and anyone attempting to engage you in the pigeon drop or bank examiner scams.
- Do not trust someone because he has a friendly voice or appears to be an authoritative figure.
- Swindlers usually are friendly and have honest faces and pleasant personalities to gain your trust and steal your money.
- **AVOID** making cash transactions in secret.
- **AVOID** making an employee a joint owner of your bank account or your property.
- Be sure the person who handles your money can be trusted.
- **AVOID** offers of assistance from strangers inside the bank or near the bank. Never accept.

November 9

- Always discuss any large transaction with your banker. Some bankers are trained to be **ALERT** and **AWARE** of bank scams.
- Be **ALERT** and **AWARE** of scams to confirm bank information whether by phone, at home, or e-mail.
- No financial institution or government agency ever uses customers to conduct internal investigations.
- Many financial institutions request that customers read and sign a form when they wish to withdraw a large amount of cash.
- The form **ALERTS** consumers to these scams and encourages them to talk to a bank or law enforcement officer if certain conditions are present. This is not an attempt to keep your money or control how it's spent. It's to protect you from fraud.
- **AVOID** giving credit cards, checkbooks, or savings account passbooks to your housekeeper or caretaker.

November 10

TELEMARKETING

Telemarketing is a common method of stealing from senior citizens. Here are several statements used in scams.

- You must act now!
- You've won a free gift or vacation.
- You can't afford to miss this no risk offer.
- Pay only postage and handling.
- You must send money, give a credit card number, a bank account number, or have a check picked up by a carrier.
- Make money at home.

November 11

OUT AND ABOUT

- Have fun, but remember *The Unique Triple A*™ strategies.
- **AVOID** walking alone at night, have a buddy system even during the daytime.
- Stay **ALERT** and be tuned-in to your surroundings.
- **AVOID** being taken by surprise.
- Be **AWARE** and prepared, even in your own neighborhood.
- Stand tall and walk confidently, don't show fear and **AVOID** looking like a victim.
- Making brief eye contact shows you are **ALERT** and **AWARE.**
- Know where you are going and how to get there.
- Stay away from vacant lots, alleys, or construction sites.
- **AVOID** dark deserted routes, even if they are the shortest.

November 12

- The way you react could be the difference between becoming a victim and **AVOIDING** a potentially dangerous encounter.

- One of the best of *The Unique Triple A*™ safety tips for seniors is to discourage someone from following through with an assault by preventing a potential confrontation in the first place.

- Although it is vital to do everything you can to **AVOID** danger and prevent a confrontation, it is also essential to realize that if an attacker is armed, the best option is to cooperate.

- There may be a loss of money or personal items, but nothing is worth risking life and limb, including your purse. **AVOID** fighting for it. Fighting for a purse with straps is dangerous.

- Use the buddy system, whenever possible.

November 13

USING ATMS

- Try to **AVOID** ATMs and go inside your bank for transactions.
- Go during daylight hours and use the buddy system. Change deposit and withdrawal routines.
- Choose a busy ATM location near populated areas, or go inside a grocery store that has ATM machines.
- Pre-plan and complete all transaction paperwork before going to ATM.
- Put your money away quickly and leave immediately. **AVOID** carrying purse.
- **AVOID** flashing your card and cash.
- If you feel uncomfortable during a transaction, stop transactions and leave.
- If someone offers to let you go ahead of him or her at the ATM machine, decline and leave.
- If someone approaches your car at the drive through ATM, roll up your window and leave.
- **AVOID** assistance from strangers.

November 14

IN YOUR CAR

- **AVOID** displaying and leaving valuables inside car.
- Keep gas tank full and engine properly maintained to **AVOID** breakdowns.
- When paying for gas whether inside station or at pump, be **ALERT** and **AWARE** your car is locked and secured. While pumping gas, take purse with you or place on car floor out of sight, or in trunk, lock all doors, close windows.
- Plan your routes and **AVOID** alleys or dark areas. Travel well-lit and busy streets. Don't enter dark parking lots or deserted garages.
- If you suspect someone is following you, drive to the nearest open public place.
- **AVOID** picking up hitchhikers.
- Always have keys in hand when approaching car, be **ALERT** and **AWARE** of surroundings, and check around, inside car before entering.

November 15

<u>Drive SMART</u>...

By the year 2030, an estimated one in five drivers in the US will be 65 or older. A healthy, responsive body and **ALERT** mind, requires good nutrition, adequate rest, and exercise to maintain or increase strength, flexibility, and sharp reflexes.

Mental exercises, such as crossword puzzles, games with words or numbers, jigsaw puzzles, charades, and solitaire involve thinking skills. For physical fitness to strengthen upper arms and hands, lift light-weight items, like soup cans, water bottles, or squeeze a small ball or stuffed animal.

Regular eye and ear exams are keys to minimize, prevent, or slow impairments. Medications may affect your ability to drive safely. Is your car the proper fit? Can you see clearly over the steering wheel? Reach the brake and accelerator with ease? Get in and out with ease?

November 16

Sharing what you know can help protect someone who you know from scams. People listen to those they trust, such as a friend. Sadly, only 1 out of 100 cases of senior fraud are reported. Scam examples:

Mystery Shopper Scam...

Someone hired by an "alleged" retail company to evaluate the quality of services in their store or restaurant. The mystery shopper (you) is directed to buy an item or order food, write a report on their experience and get reimbursed. Be **ALERT**:

- Advertises under "help wanted" in newspaper or email.
- Mandates you pay a fee to be "certified."
- Asks you to deposit their "fake" check in your bank account.

Sweetheart Scam...

Love is blind! Scammers' frequent chat rooms, online dating websites, social media. After a time of courting, they say they are in love with you and ask to wire her/him emergency cash or to buy a ticket to come see you.

November 17

AT HOME

- Your first line of defense around your home is to keep the outside premises well lit at night, and keep curtains or blinds closed.

- Consider electronic surveillance systems, alarm systems, and/or a dog to enhance your home security.

- When you go out, make your home sound and appear occupied by using an automatic timer to turn on interior lights and a radio or TV.

- Be **ALERT** and **AWARE,** day and night, leaving drapes completely open is an opportunity for criminals to observe your movements, routines, and valuables.

- Use only your first initial in phone books, directories, and apartment lobbies.

- If you live alone, don't advertise it.

- Keep your garage doors locked and secured.

November 18

- Be **AWARE** not to rely on security door chains when opening door. A determined assailant can easily break them. Get solid deadbolt locks as the primary source for security.
- Install and use a peephole. Install a solid wood door with solid deadbolt locks.
- **AVOID** leaving notes on the door when going out.
- **AVOID** hiding keys under the mat, flowerpot, atop a doorframe or other conspicuous places.
- Protect windows and other points of entry with good locks (see August), or other security devices (such as a length of wooden doweling placed in a track to prevent a window or sliding glass door from opening).
- Mark/engrave and record your personal property with a secret identification number.
- Keep bonds, stock certificates, seldom worn jewelry, and stamp and coin collections in a safe deposit box.

November 19

- **AVOID** keeping large amounts of cash at home.
- Use direct deposit for social security, pension checks or other monthly sources of income.
- Keep emergency numbers for police and fire agencies handy.
- Post medication/prescription and medical information on refrigerator for emergency personnel (http://www.vialoflife.com).
- **Be ALERT** and never open your door unless you know the person.
- If someone comes to your door with an emergency (for example, a traffic accident or an injury), **AVOID** and do not let them into your house! Call 9-1-1 for them!
- If a stranger asks for help to use your phone, offer to place the call instead. **AVOID** letting them inside.

November 20

PUBLIC TRANSPORTATION

- When using a bus or subway, plan your route.
- Stay **ALERT** and **AWARE** while waiting for transportation.
- Be **ALERT** and **AWARE** if you sit on a bus bench - who is behind you? Stay awake.
- Wait near the attendant's stand if possible in subways.
- **AVOID** carrying a purse if you can.
- Use a fanny pack, not a purse with straps.
- Attempt to sit near the driver.
- Keep your belongings in your lap, snug to body, not on the seat next to you or on shoulder.
- Use busy, well-lit transportation stops.
- Be **ALERT** and **AWARE** who gets on or off the bus or trolley with you.
- If you feel you are being followed or harassed, advise the driver.

November 21

SHOPPING

- **AVOID** carrying packages that block your view and are too heavy.
- **AVOID** carrying more cash, credit cards, and checks than necessary. **AVOID** flashing cash and other tempting targets such as expensive jewelry.
- Wear a fanny pack and **AVOID** using a purse with straps.
- Keep wallet in an inside jacket or front pants pocket.
- Make sure someone is **AWARE** where you're going and when you expect to return.
- Wear comfortable clothes and shoes.
- If a friend or a taxi takes you home, ask them to wait and be **ALERT** and **AWARE** until you are safely inside.
- Have your car or house key in hand as you approach your vehicle or home.

November 22

SOLICITORS: DOOR-TO-DOOR, PHONE

- Hang up immediately if harassing or obscene phone calls.

- If the caller persists, call law enforcement and the phone company.

- Be **ALERT, AWARE** by using a Caller ID or blocked call services to **AVOID** phone solicitors and screen calls.

- **AVOID** giving personal information and credit card information over phone.

- **AVOID** and never open the door to someone you do not know.

- Always be **ALERT** and use the peephole or window for observation.

November 23

- Teach grandchildren what to do when strangers come to the home. Teach them how to use the phone, and how to call for help.
- Tell them to **AVOID** answering the door and speaking to a solicitor.
- **AVOID** getting into a conversation with a solicitor through the door. They will try to converse with you, but getting into a conversation of any kind with a solicitor only encourages them to stay and attempt to enter. Learn to say no.
- If solicitors try to approach you while you are outside, **AVOID** their approach. Wave them off and say no. Walk back into your house, close and lock your door. Call police if they do not leave.
- Observe where the solicitor goes next and notice what they do. Look for suspicious behavior such as looking in car windows, testing doors for locks, or entering back yards.

November 24

- Be **ALERT** and **AWARE** of burglars who attempt to get your attention at the front of your house while the partner goes to the back to gain entry.
- Call your neighbors and warn them to also watch for the suspicious activity.
- If you notice anything suspicious, please call the police department when the activity is happening.
- Working together with neighbors, not opening the doors, and monitoring a solicitor's behavior is the best way to reduce the risk for soliciting-related crime.

November 25

ELDER ABUSE

AWARENESS will enable you to help yourself, friends, or family members who may be in trouble. By being **ALERT** to situations that could lead to abuse of an elderly person, you may be able to prevent a serious injury or save a life. Be on the **ALERT** if you don't hear from elderly friends for several days, stop by and check on them. If you observe any of the following, notify the proper authorities.

- Look for any unusual, unexplained bumps, bruises, or cuts. Look for unusual changes in behavior. Be **ALERT to** salesmen at the house or suspicious cars in driveway. If elderly friends tell you about someone inappropriately spending their money, report it to the police. Be **AWARE** if elderly friends' homes are unusually unkempt or filthy. Be **AWARE** if they begin to look malnourished, or if they are not receiving proper medication.

November 26

CRIMES IN CONVALESCENT HOMES

Be ALERT And AWARE Of These Signs Of Abuse...

Emotional/Psychological Abuse: Verbal threats of punishment, constant harassment, threat of withdrawal of services.

Financial: Theft of personal effects, overcharging for services, fraudulent billing for non-services.

Neglect: Dehydration, malnutrition, bedsores, rashes, sores, lice, untreated medical condition, over or under medicated.

Physical: Rough handling or grabbing, hitting or slapping, dragging the patient by the arms or hair, lack of physical activity.

Sexual Assault: When a senior is forced, manipulated, coerced into unwanted sexual activity, or the senior lacks the ability to consent to any sexual activity.

November 27

In Looking For A Convalescent Home...

- Be **ALERT** and **AWARE** of the surroundings.
- Check inside and outside of the home for cleanliness and grounds if well kept.
- When walking inside, smell the air. It should smell clean and fresh, not musty or have a high chemical smell which can indicate overall concern by the caretakers for cleanliness.
- Talk to employees about the condition of the home and their work environment, their attitude, concerns about the quality of the job they perform.
- Look at the home's equipment to make sure it is in good working condition and not outdated.
- Be **ALERT** to research for complaints, fines with local Ombudsman.

November 28

Be **ALERT** and **AWARE** that often convalescent home crimes and related quality of life issues go unreported for the following reasons:

- Fear retaliation from their caretakers for reporting crimes.
- Feel that the crimes committed against them are just a fact of life and nothing that can be done to change them.
- Thinks that no one cares about them or what happens to them.
- Embarrassed to tell family or friends because of what their family or friends might think.
- Ashamed to ask their family or friends for assistance.
- Convalescent employees who witnessed a crime may not report these crimes, in fear of retaliation from their employer.

November 29

GOBBLE OF THANKS FOR GOOD HEALTH

Eye Care...

Cataracts are a clouding of the lens inside the eye and usually develop very gradually until the vision is impacted, and are one of the leading causes of vision loss. Smoking, excessive alcohol use, and diabetes can increase the formation of cataracts. Wearing a hat and sunglasses to block sunlight, and good nutrition may help to delay cataracts forming. An important step are regular eye exams to help identify cataracts early in order to work out a treatment plan.

Live SMART. Smart living includes eating green leafy vegetables and other foods rich in antioxidants that can help reduce the risk of cataracts. **AVOID** spreading germs to the eye and face area by washing hands thoroughly and often.

Next Eye Care Appointment...

November 30

Medications...

Manage your medications. Make sure you understand the exact dosage and timing for each prescription. If you have more than one doctor, make sure each one knows what medications you are taking, including over-the-counter drugs. Always ask if there is a generic available. A name brand medication can cost 10 times what generics cost. Generic drugs are chemically identical to their brand name counterparts and just as effective. Ordering a higher dose of scored pills that can be split in half can yield significant savings.

Whether you have a medical condition or not, it is imperative that first responders KNOW your medical and emergency information! Obtain emergency medical information forms from local fire departments and organizations such as the Vial of Life program. Complete and affix on refrigerator. (Refer to EMERGENCY INFORMATION and MEDICATION FORMS).

BONUS SAFETY TIP

Tips For The Disabled...

One of the best safety tips to discourage someone from following through with an assault, is to **AVOID** a potential confrontation in the first place.

When shopping, use the buddy system as there is safety in numbers.

Be realistic about your limitations. **AVOID** places or situations that put you at risk, such as dark alleys and unlit parking lots.

Be **ALERT** before you carry any type of non-lethal weapon (pepper spray, Taser), and take a course in these weapons and/or a self-defense class for seniors/disabled. Some classes teach how to turn items commonly carried (see WEAPONS), as well as walking canes into weapons.

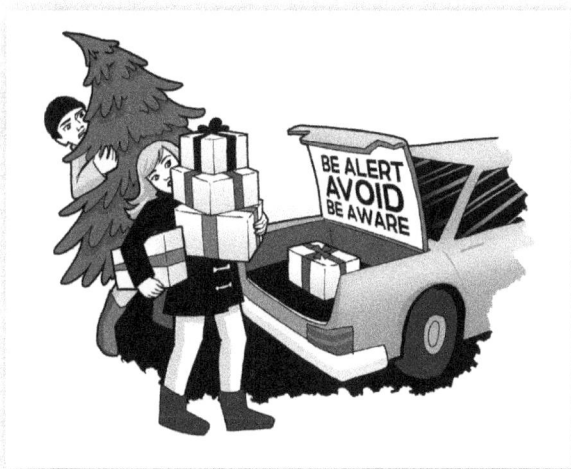

December

JOLLY SAFETY

———

Shop 'til You Drop

December 1

CHARITY FRAUD

Be **AWARE** there will be many charities collecting donations throughout the holiday season by phone, door-to-door, at shopping areas, and on the street.

Be **ALERT** to research before you donate and that the organization you donate to is a reputable and legitimate charity.

- Each state, city, and county government has a set of ordinances before issuing a solicitation license to charitable organizations. Check the validity of a charity on the state's Attorney General's web site, the National Charities Information Bureau (NCIB), the Better Business Bureau at http://www.give.org, or National Crime Prevention Council at www.ncpc.org

December 2

- Take the time to learn about the charitable organization you support or are considering supporting.
- The IRS governs non-profits with ordinance codes: 501(c) (3) for non-profit organizations (proceeds or monies raised go directly to the charitable organization), and a profit organization working for a non-profit organization that may take some of the proceeds or monies gained from any event held for a specific organization and pay for costs, while the rest of the income goes to the charitable organization.
- Read and understand everything before you donate.
- Ask every charity solicitor who solicits money from you where and how your contribution will be used.

December 3

- Be **ALERT** to ask for the charity's tax-exempt letter indicating its IRS status. You can't claim a tax-deductible donation if the charity does not have one.
- Never give cash. Make all donations by check to the organization, or use employee-withholding programs through your work. Keep all records.
- A charity DOES NOT NEED your social security number.

Red Flags For The Following Signs...

- Pressure to sign blank checks, or donations of substantial amounts, to organizations you have not checked out.
- Unwillingness to explain what the organization is about, or where your money or gift will be going.

December 4

- Tricky wording on issues you don't understand.
- A telephone call with a high-pressure appeal or a mailing that promises free stuff in exchange for a donation.
- Take your time to investigate these organizations, and tell the solicitor whether in person or over the telephone that you would like to do some research on the charity/organization.
- Always ask for a name and call back number and be **ALERT** if they don't give one in return, or say they will call you back.

Questionable And/Or Illegal...

- Prize offers.
- Spam e-mail.
- Chain letters.
- Unsolicited gifts, usually tokens enclosed in direct mail solicitations.

December 5

CREDIT REPAIR FRAUD

- Be **AWARE** and **AVOID** solicitations that remove damaging information from your credit score. These scam artists claim they can get truthful information removed from your credit report for a fee, which is false.
- Always check through credit reporting agencies for errors, updated data, and how to repair credit.
- Some nonprofit organizations can help you rebuild your credit at no cost.

December 6

ONLINE SHOPPING

"Black Friday" and "Cyber Monday" means many of you will log on and click your way through hundreds of cybermalls looking for massive holiday sales and huge deals. Be **AWARE** there's a Grinch ready to steal your jingle and your joy.

- Be **ALERT** and **AWARE** to **AVOID** "phishing" and other suspicious related schemes/scams. Opening a contaminated link may lead you to a phishing website where shoppers who click through are redirected to a fraudulent site designed to steal your identity and your cash. Examine the website's URL. Shoppers should always look in the address box for the "s" in https:// and in the lower-right corner for the "lock" symbol before paying.
- **AVOID** unsolicited spam e-mails and phishing websites.

December 7

- **AVOID** giving out any personal information to anyone soliciting through online and phone calls, especially when asked for social security, bank account, and/or credit card numbers.
- **AVOID** "act quickly" or sense of urgency ads.
- Be **ALERT** to online auctions or bids.
- **AVOID** giving out social security number.
- Be **AWARE** that the Fair Credit Billing Act covers only credit card purchases, not debit card purchases. **AVOID** using your debit card for online purchases. A debit card is just like cash and if compromised, your bank account can be wiped out.
- If you have received a scam e-mail, please notify the IC3 by filing a complaint at htpp://www.ic3.gov

December 8

A KEY TO GETTING STROKELESS

Hackers, Identity Theft, Passwords...

- **AVOID** using keyboard to type passwords. Go "strokeless." In one of your flash drive documents, type in a title to a song, phrase, or a movie. Example: *Master and Commander: The Far Side of the World*. Take the first letter from each word (mactfsotw), type them somewhere in a document (also add symbols or numbers). COPY and PASTE into your log in.

- Change your passwords often. Update online accounts (bank, credit cards), with strong passwords that consist of lower and uppercase letters, numbers, and symbols. Use a unique password for EACH account with the keyless stroke method.

- Obtain a copy of your credit report. Read carefully for any suspicious activities, fraudulent transactions, or accounts listed. Dispute errors by contacting the credit reporting firms as well as the businesses involved.

December 9

- **AVOID** sharing your passwords with anyone or revealing the answers to your security questions. Thoroughly shred documents containing personal information before disposing.
- Be **AWARE** cell phones can be easily stolen and provide all your sensitive information.
- Never enter your credit card number, user identification, or password without the "s" and "lock" symbol.
- **AVOID** using your debit card for online purchases. A debit card is just like cash and if compromised, your bank account can be wiped out.
- Always log off after an online banking session.

December 10

HEAD ABOVE CLOUDS?

- The cloud is a convenient place to store files and access them from any device, but it can be hacked like the fluffy cloud it is.
- Use a complex password or "copy and paste" your strokeless password. Use different passwords for each account. Be **ALERT** you can enable two-step verification with a special code sent to your phone to access your service.
- Turn off automatic backups.
- Don't upload anything you don't want to end up on TMZ.
- For safe online shopping, ensure your apps are downloaded from a trusted source, such as the Android Market, Apple App Store, or the Amazon App Store.
- When you download the app, it will ask for various permissions, so be **ALERT** to read through them, note whether they make sense (does a shopping app need access to your contact list?). Choose apps with a high rating.

December 11

Connection Protection...

- Your computer should always have the most recent updates installed for spam filters, anti-virus, and anti-spyware software, and a secure firewall.
- Webroot found that only 40 percent of respondents have a security app installed on their smartphones and tablets, putting their devices and personal information at risk.

December 12

AT HOME

- **AVOID** displaying your tree and gifts in an open window with drapes wide open.
- **AVOID** posting your complete name on your mailbox or on your house. A burglar can call directory assistance to get your telephone number and call your home while in front of your house to confirm if you are away.
- Indoor and outdoor lights should be on automatic timers.
- Be **ALERT** about locking doors and windows when you leave the house, even for a few minutes.
- When setting up a Christmas tree or other holiday display, make sure doors and passageways are clear inside your home.
- Be **ALERT** your tree is mounted on a sturdy base.

December 13

- Be **ALERT** that tree light wirings are not damaged or frayed (can cause a fire).
- Place tree in water or wet sand to keep green.
- Never place wrapping paper in fireplace.
- **AVOID** leaving descriptive telephone machine messages that describe your holiday "time away" dates (see vacation tips in July).
- **AVOID** comments about items you've purchased or received as gifts on social media.

After Christmas Day...

- **AVOID** piling up empty gift boxes from new expensive valuables (computer, TV), in front of your house for trash collection.
- Burglars appreciate knowing that you have expensive gifts inside for them to steal. Break the boxes down or cut them up and throw inside trash container, not outside of container.

December 14

On the first day of Christmas, you can prevent crime by keeping your car safe from break-ins and thefts.

SHOPPING

Parking Before Shopping...

- If you must shop at night, use buddy system and park in a well-lighted area as close to the stores as possible. Take notice of where you parked. Be **ALERT** and **AWARE**. Keep your full attention on your surroundings.

- Be **ALERT** and **AWARE** of isolated areas, such as subterranean parking lots, dimly lit areas, and subterranean parking columns/walls.

- Keep your vehicle's doors locked and windows closed. Keep your car inside clean to **AVOID** someone hiding under anything. **AVOID** parking next to vans, trucks with camper shells, or cars with tinted windows.

- **AVOID** purchasing from anyone selling in the parking lot or out of their vehicle. Be **AWARE** of the "rock in the box" scam. You'll get rocks, not the item.

December 15

On the second day of Christmas, you can prevent crime by dressing casually and comfortably.

The Unique Triple A™ brand logo consists of a large brim hat and high heels to illustrate some of the objects that can block your view and freedom of movement to defend yourself. Expensive jewelry attracts the wrong kind of attention. Being **ALERT** and **AWARE** helps to **AVOID** potential dangerous situations while shopping. Be **AWARE** of other objects and distractions while shopping.

- **AVOID** overloading yourself with packages that block your view and freedom of movement to defend yourself properly and **AVOID** mishaps. You will be too concerned in balancing/struggling with the packages and not be **ALERT** and **AWARE** of your surroundings and individuals.
- Dress casually and comfortably.
- Men, be **AWARE** and **ALERT** of *The Unique Triple A*™ safety precautions to **AVOID** your wallet being taken.

December 16

On the third day of Christmas, you can prevent crime by keeping your information safe and secure.

- **AVOID** buying more than you can carry. Plan ahead and take a friend with you, or ask a store employee/escort to help you carry packages to car.
- **AVOID** wearing expensive jewelry. **AVOID** carrying a purse with straps, if possible.
- **AVOID** talking on a cell phone when walking through parking lots and streets. Your cell phone itself can be a tempting target to thieves, as well as eliminating your **ALERTNESS** and **AWARENESS.**
- **AVOID** flashing large amounts of cash or offering tempting targets for theft such as expensive jewelry or clothing.
- **AVOID** carrying unnecessary cash, credit cards, or checks. Carry only what you need for that shopping day and use a credit card rather than a debit card to stop payments quickly in the event of a problem or refunds.

December 17

On the fourth day of Christmas, you can prevent crime by reporting suspicious behavior to store security.

- Shop before dark whenever possible.
- Coordinate shopping trips with a friend.
- Stay **ALERT** and **AWARE** of your surroundings, packages, and personal items. Walk with authority, always making eye contact with others.
- Beware of strangers approaching you for any reason. Con artists may try various methods of distracting you with the intention of taking your money or belongings.
- Consider alternate options to pay for your merchandise, such as one time or multiuse disposable credit cards or money orders.
- **For Your Checks Only**. Use first name initial. If you have a post office box, list it on your checks. Don't forget to do the same with your driver's license and car registration forms.

December 18

On the fifth day of Christmas, you can prevent crime by protecting your valuables.

- Be **ALERT** and wait until ready to pay before taking out your credit card or checkbook. An enterprising thief can shoulder surf to get your account information while you are "displaying" your information. Whisper phone number to the clerk, when asked.
- Be extra careful if you do carry a wallet or purse. They are the prime targets of criminals in crowded shopping areas, transportation terminals, bus stops, on buses, and other rapid transit.
- Deter pickpockets. If you carry a purse, carry close to your body (shorter straps to prevent dangling), and put wallet inside a coat or front trouser pocket (use comb trick). Purchase RFID products to protect ID.
- Be **ALERT, AWARE** of your packages, purses, wallets, and valuables at all times.
- Remember to **AVOID** crowded transportation, elevators, or crowded lines whenever possible.

December 19

On the sixth day of Christmas, you can prevent crime by talking to children about stranger danger.

- If possible, leave small children at home with a trusted person. Teach children to stay close to you at all times while shopping. However, teach them to go to a store clerk and ask for help in case they are separated from you. Tell them to immediately tell you if a stranger bothers them.
- **AVOID** children going to restroom alone.
- Teach children their full name, address, and telephone number to give to police
- Children should never be allowed to go to the car alone, and never left alone in the car.

December 20

On the seventh day of Christmas, you can prevent crime by keeping valuables and gifts out of sight in trunk.

Returning To Car...

If you are ready to leave the mall and feel uneasy about entering the parking lot or garage by yourself, stay in the mall and ask for a security escort. If you believe you are in danger, call 9-1-1 immediately.

- Have your keys in hand when approaching your car.
- Be **AWARE** of suspicious people near your car, loitering, or approaching you. **AVOID** solicitors or anyone asking for time or distracting you.
- Upon approaching your car, be **ALERT** and **AWARE**. Scan the area and your car from a distance. Look around your car, under it, and rear seat before entering. Look for signs of pry marks around doors and windows. Are your doors still locked? Are there large columns nearby that can hide a person?

December 21

On the eighth day of Christmas, you can prevent crime with car keys.

- Be **ALERT,** don't electronically unlock your car until you are within view of your car to **AVOID** a thief from getting into the car and waiting to strike when you least expect it.
- **AVOID** fumbling for car keys. Have them in the defense position between your fingers before approaching your car. Use the panic button on your key fob to activate car alarm and lights for help.
- Be **ALERT** and do not linger to sort packages.
- After entering your car, lock, secure it immediately, and leave.
- If you return to your car and find a van or occupied car next to it, return to the store for assistance. Be **ALERT** and **AWARE** of your instincts and **AVOID** being a possible victim.

December 22

On the ninth day of Christmas, you can prevent crime by being a safe driver on the road.

DRIVING

- **AVOID** driving at night if possible during the holiday rush. If you must shop at night, park in a well-lighted area and use the buddy system.
- Keep all car doors locked and windows closed while in or out of your car. Set your alarm and/or also use an anti-theft device.
- Lock your packages and gifts in trunk. Do not leave packages visible in your car.
- **AVOID** leaving packages, purse, or valuables on the seat of your car. This creates a temptation for thieves. If you must leave something in the car, lock it in the trunk or put it out of sight.
- Be **ALERT** and **AWARE** when stopped at signals or stop signs. Check your rearview mirror to be **AWARE** if anyone is following you. **AVOID** going home if you feel you are, and drive to open businesses or any 24-hour emergency facility.

December 23

On the tenth day of Christmas, you can prevent crime by recognizing danger and taking action.

One of the best holiday gifts you can give to yourself is to become **AWARE,** and to equip yourself to live securely and as comfortably as you can. Karate or other form of self-defense is one means of protection. However, safety starts with **ALERTNESS**. In martial arts, you must become proficient in offensive skills, such as coordination, balance, strength, agility, and being able to strike targets, such as eyes and noses.

The three skilled gifts of *The Unique Triple A*™ for yourself can minimize physical techniques and fighting.

- **ALERTNESS** can help eliminate potential dangers.
- **AWARENESS** is recognizing threats with forethought and common sense.
- **AVOIDING** dangers requires no physical techniques or fighting.

December 24

On the eleventh day of Christmas, you can prevent crime by getting home from a party safely.

Out on the town at office parties and holiday celebrations, you'll find pubs, restaurants, and other venues are often crowded.

- **AVOID** leaving purse over the back of your chair. Keep purse and wallet close to your body to **AVOID** pickpockets.
- Busy places make it easier for the sneak thief, so be **ALERT** at all times.
- **AVOID** any potential disturbances on the street. Stay with friends.
- **AVOID** drinking too much which dulls all your senses.
- Dress sensibly and comfortably.

"What do you call people who are afraid of Santa Claus? Claustrophobic."

~ ANONYMOUS

December 25

On the twelfth day of Christmas, you can prevent crime by keeping your home safe from break-ins and thefts.

GIFTS

- With an engraving tool, engrave bikes, electronics with your ID number or driver's license number. **AVOID** using social security number. Record make, model, and serial number for insurance purposes.
- If the item is stolen, and later recovered by police, the engraved number will allow investigators to get property back to you.
- **AVOID** displaying gifts in a window or a doorway.
- Properly dispose of gift packaging and boxes by breaking up cartons and placing them in garbage bags. This can **AVOID** advertising what you received so that thieves can't "gift" themselves with your gifts.

December 26

Start making resolutions for the upcoming New Year.

Begin the countdown for new beginnings of a happy, healthy, and safer New Year!

December 27

To Launch and Organize to help clean and repair your local parks. Be **ALERT** and **AWARE** of play equipment that needs repair, or has been vandalized, and report to city or county parks and recreation staff. Residents should continue to work with local government to maintain neighborhood parks.

December 28

GET SET

4

To Clean Up. Tired of talking about the disarray in the neighborhood? Instead, get involved with the neighborhood and start a clean-up. Involve everyone — teens, children, senior citizens. Litter, abandoned cars, and run-down buildings tell criminals that you don't care about where you live or each other. Call the city public works department and ask for help in cleaning up. It is their responsibility as well.

December 29

3

Aim You Goals. Rise. Volunteer in your community to make a difference.

December 30

GO

2

With the New Year approaching, safety resolutions should consist of personal development. Every improvement of your life always comes from CHANGE that leads to a MINDSET of opportunities, skills, and knowledge for CONFIDENCE. With CONFIDENCE comes COMPETENCE, which is a commitment of extraordinarily prepared behavior, self-assurance, and attitude in what you think and do. That is *The Unique Triple A*™ WISDOM for body, soul, and mind.

December 31

CELEBRATE

1

Believing in yourself and knowing you are prepared mentally are effective skills. Celebrate the New Year safely and responsibly. Don't fire guns into the air. People involved in celebrating by firing guns into the air do not realize the dangers posed by their actions. **AVOID** being with anyone involved in this. If you're arrested for shooting a gun into the air, you will be prosecuted to the fullest extent of the law.

BONUS SAFETY TIP

Holidays, such as Christmas and the New Year are busy times of the year for almost everyone, including the criminal, and most people can be vulnerable to being victimized through criminal activities.

Law enforcement agencies nationwide rely on our involvement in crime prevention to make an impact on personal safety and crime every day. Preventing crime is always preferable to reacting after a crime.

If you see a crime being committed, or believe crime is occurring in your neighborhood, call the police. **AVOID** taking the law into your own hands. If you own a gun and possess the appropriate training and permits, always be **ALERT** and **AWARE** about using and firing them if you think a burglar is IN your home.

Color Codes of Awareness

COLOR CODES OF AWARENESS

Used by law enforcement, military, and martial arts the Cooper Color Codes describes your state of mind and observations in color zones. How inattentive and oblivious are you in your work environment, or any environment, day in and day out? You can be stupid, inattentive, and oblivious and get away with it until you happen to be surprised by an attacker or opportunist.

White Zone: Lowest level. You are relaxed, unaware, not **ALERT**, not prepared, walking around head down, and daydreaming. "He came out of nowhere," or "I didn't see him."

Yellow Zone: Relaxed state of general **ALERTNESS.** In this zone, you use your eyes and ears to monitor and assess your surroundings, and carry yourself in a way that others know you are **AWARE** of everything. When your mental radar picks up something, you immediately escalate one level up on the scale, Orange.

Orange Zone: Heightened state of **ALERTNESS.** You have a focal point that brought your attention, a possible or potential dangerous situation or person. Now that you are **AWARE**, you are prepared to leave, run, or escalate to the highest level, Red.

Red Zone: You think strategy, mentally prepare to fight. You are looking for an avenue of escape, keys in hand for defense, and you know what you are going to do. The key is that you were mentally prepared for a conflict if the situation demanded. Your main enemy is reaction time. If you are not **AWARE** of your surroundings, and fail to see the potential danger or person, he may overwhelm you before you can react effectively.

Remove criminal opportunities and you can remove the risks to you. If you should find yourself faced with a life-threatening attack, you will be faced by three enormous difficulties. They are:

1. Recognizing the presence of the predator in time.
2. Realizing, internalizing, and accepting that THAT PERSON, RIGHT THERE, is about to harm or kill you for reasons you do not understand.
3. Overcoming your reluctance to do lethal violence against a fellow human being.

Glossary

These criminal law definitions were summarized from the California Penal Code and may vary in other states or countries.

Assault. An unlawful attempt, coupled with a present ability, to commit a violent injury on the person of another; violent physical or verbal attack; to rape; sexual assault.

Assault & Battery. Battery is the unlawful application of physical force; requires no minimum degree of force.

Bank Examiner. A scheme when con artists pose as either law enforcement or a bank official pretending to need your help to conduct an investigation. You are asked to withdraw your money and hand it over as they promise to redeposit it or return the money after they complete their investigation. Of course, you will never see your money again.

Burglary. Illegal entry into a building or vehicle for the purposes of committing an offense.

Burner Phones. Pay as you go or pre-paid phones with a different number. Good to use to maintain private phone number when giving out a contact number.

C.E.R.T. Community Emergency Response Team refers to community volunteers who receive specific training in basic disaster response skills. May take different names.

CPTED. Crime Prevention Through Environmental Design is a multi-disciplinary approach to deterring criminal behavior through environmental design of buildings, ranging from landscape to restrooms.

Identity Theft. A form of stealing someone's identity in which someone pretends to be someone else, by assuming that person's identity, and gain access to financial funds.

Phishing. The act of attempting to acquire information, such as passwords and credit card details by masquerading as a trustworthy entity in an electronic communication, such as social media, websites, e-mails, and instant messaging.

Pigeon Drop Scam. Con artists work in pairs or teams. One befriends the victim (called the pigeon), while the other approaches the victim with money or valuables he claims to have just found. The two crooks engage in a rehearsed conversation with the victim to agree to split and share the found money among them. The con artists will "arrange" to meet at a lawyer's office or somewhere else of their choosing. They want to trust you and will ask you to put up some "good faith" money of the share, which they will return to you after they split the money. They will even go to the bank with you while you withdraw money. Later, when you arrive at their designated spot, they are gone with your money.

RFID. Radio Frequency Identification technology are chips inside most ID cards (credit/debit, license, passport), that allow someone to wave card in front of a scanner vs. a magnetic strip by wireless use of electromagnetic fields for automatic identification. Stores personal information. Criminals can "skim" these cards for identity theft. Shielding products, such as metal-lined or aluminum shielding wallets, purses can help block skimming.

Robbery. Taking of personal property from the possession of another, from his person or immediate presence, and against his/her will, accomplished by means of force or fear.

Theft. In which property belonging to another is taken without that person's consent; sometimes used synonymously with larceny; the intent to deprive the rightful owner of it.

Resources

Please note that at the time of print, resources were accurate, but subject to change. Check occasionally for updates or changes.

BABY CHILD CARE

National Center on Shaken Baby Syndrome
2955 Harrison Boulevard, Suite 102
Ogden, UT 84403
1.888.273.0071
http://www.dontshake.com

TRUSTLINE
California's Background Check for In-Home Childcare.
1.800.822.8490

BULLYING

- http://www.stopbullyingnow.com
- http://www.nces.ed.gov
- http://www.stopbullying.gov

CAMPUS SECURITY

Clergy Center for Security on Campus
Nonprofit organization for prevention of campus crime.
110 Gallagher Road
Wayne, PA 19087
1.484.580.8754
http://www.clergycenter.org

CRIME PREVENTION

National Crime Prevention Council
Private, nonprofit organization helping people, seniors, families, and their communities stay safe from crime, and promote crime prevention.
2001 Jefferson Davis Highway, Suite 901
Arlington, VA 22202
1.202.466.6272

DOMESTIC VIOLENCE

National Coalition Against Domestic Violence
A national information and referral center for the general public, battered women and their children, and allied and member agencies and organizations.
One Broadway, Suite 210 B
Denver, CO 80203
1.303.839.1852

National Domestic Violence Hotline
A phone counselor can help guide you through the process of safely leaving a relationship.
http://www.thehotline.org
1.800.799.SAFE (7233)

National Network to End Domestic Violence
1400 16th Street, NW, Suite 400
Washington, DC 20036
1.202.543.5566

Men and Domestic Violence
http://www.helpguide.org

NO MORE
NO MORE is a public awareness and engagement campaign focused on ending domestic violence and sexual assault. NO MORE is aligned with hundreds of organizations working at the local, state and national levels on prevention, advocacy, and services for survivors. In partnership, Joyful Heart Foundation is to heal, educate and empower survivors.
http://www.nomore.org
http://www.joyfulheartfoundation.org

DRUNK DRIVERS

Mothers Against Drunk Driving (MADD)
Organization of victims and non-victims determined to make a difference in the lives of those victimized by impaired driving crashes.
511 East John Carpenter Freeway, Suite 700
Irving, TX 75062
1.877. MADD.HELP or 1.877.623.3435

Students Against Destructive Decisions (SADD) formerly Students Against Drunk Drivers
Providing students "with the best prevention and intervention tools possible to deal with the issues of underage drinking, other drug use, impaired driving, and other destructive decisions."
255 Main Street
Marlborough, MA 01752
1.877.SADD.INC
http://www.sadd.org

SCAMS/FRAUD/CREDIT INFO

Equifax Credit Information Services, Inc.
P.O. Box 105873
Atlanta, GA 30348
1.800.685.1111: Credit Report Inquiries.
1.888.766.0008: Place Fraud Alert on Your Credit.
1.866.493.9788: Credit Reports, Scores, Identity Theft.
1.888.202.4025: Business Solutions.
http://www.Equifax.com

Experian®
P.O. Box 2104
Allen, Texas 75013-3742
1.866.431.3471
1.888.397.3742: Credit Report, Dispute Information, Fraud & Identity Theft.
1.877.284.7942: Triple Advantage Credit Monitoring.
http://www.experian.com

Trans Union
P.O. Box 390
Springfield, PA 19064-390
1.800.493.2392: Credit Monitoring Service Inquires.
1.800.888.4213: Purchase a Credit Report or Get Free Annual Report.
1.800.916.8800: Dispute Items on Credit Report.
1.800.680.7289: Fraud Alerts and Identity Theft Info.
1.866.922.2100: Business Services Assistance.
http://www.TransUnion.com

Federal Trade Commission (FTC)
1.877.FTC.HELP or 1.877.382.4357
http://www.ftc.gov/complaint
http://www.consumer.ftcgov/articles

Adult Protective Services (APS)

An agency to help elder adults (65 years and older), and dependent adults (18-64 who are disabled), who are unable to meet their own needs, or are victims of abuse, neglect, or exploitation. Investigates reports of elder abuse and dependent adults who live in private homes, hotels, hospitals, and health clinics when the abuser is not a staff member. Report abuse also to law enforcement.

http://www.cdss.gov/aged

American Association of Homes, Resources & Services for the Aging

2519 Connecticut Avenue NW
Washington, DC 20008
1. 202.783.2242
http://www. hospaa.org

American Association of Retired Persons (AARP)

601 E Street, NW
Washington DC 20049
Toll-Free Nationwide:1.888.OUR.AARP (1.888.687.2277)
Toll-Free TTY: 1.877.434.7598
Toll-Free Spanish: 1.877.342.2277
International Calls: +1.202.434.3525
http://www.aarp.org

Area Agency on Aging

http://www.areaagency.org

California Association of Area Agencies on Aging (C4A)
Advocate for meeting the needs of seniors and adults with disabilities, with the purpose to implement the provisions and intent of the Older Americans Act and the Older Californians Act.
980 Ninth Street
Sacramento, California, 95814
1.916.443.2800
http://www.c4a.info

California Department of Aging
1300 National Drive, Suite 200
Sacramento, CA 95834-1992
1.916.419.7500
TDD: 800.735.2929
http://www.aging.ca.gov

National Association of Area Agencies on Aging (n4a)
1730 Rhode Island Avenue, NW, Suite 1200
Washington, DC 20036
1.202.872.0888
http://www.n4a.org

National Aging Resource Center
810 First Street, N.E. Suite 500
Washington D.C. 20002
1.202.682.2470

National Center on Elder Abuse Administration on Aging
Resource center for professionals and advocates involved in the prevention and response to elder abuse.
University of California, Irvine
101 The City Drive South, Suite 835, Rt. 81, ZC 1150
Orange, CA 92568
1.855.500.3537

National Institute on Aging
8600 Rockville Pike
Bethesda, MD 20894
1.888.346.3656 TDD 1.800.735.2258
http://www.nia.nih.gov

Ombudsman
Investigates abuse in a nursing home, board and care home, assisted living facilities and similar adult care facilities, or at a long term care facility. Administered by the California Department of Aging to bring about changes at the local, state and national levels that will improve residents' care and quality of life.
Administration for Community Living
Washington, DC 20201
Public Inquiries: 1.202.619.0724
Eldercare Locator (to find local resources): 1.800.677.1116
Email: aclinfo@acl.hhs.gov
http://www.aoa.gov

U.S. Department of Health & Human Services
200 Independence Avenue SW
Washington, DC 20201
1.877.696.6775
http://www.hhs.gov

Federal Trade Commission
If you suspect your identity has been stolen.
1.877.ID.THEFT or 1.877.438.4338

SEXUAL ASSAULTS

Rape, Abuse, and Incest National Network (RAINN)
Largest anti-sexual assault organization. Publicizes the hotline's free, confidential services. RAINN operates the National Sexual Assault Online Hotline at 1.800.656.HOPE and the National Sexual Assault Online Hotline at http://www.www.rainn.org

National Teen Dating Abuse Hotline
If you are a teen, talk to a trusted adult, such as your parents, family friend, or school counselor. You can also call the National Teen Dating Abuse Hotline, toll-free. National Teen Dating Abuse Helpline was launched in 2007 by the National Domestic Violence Hotline. This 24-hour national Web-based and telephone resource was created to help teens and young adults experiencing dating abuse, and is the only helpline in the country serving all 50 states, Puerto Rico and the Virgin Islands.
1.866.331.9474
http://www.loveisrespect.org

YWCA (Young Women's Christian Association)
A voice for women to empower. Advocacy intervention for victims and survivors. Counseling, crisis intervention, prevention education on issues, such as domestic violence.
YWCA USA National Office
2025 M Street NW, Suite 550, Washington, DC 20036
1.202.467.0801
Fax: 1.202.467.0802
http://www.ywca.org

SUICIDE/DEPRESSION

Suicide Prevention Center
Get help for yourself, deaf, loss survivors, attempt survivors, vets, and bullying, 24/7. Ayuda en España.
1.800.273.TALK (8255)

SURVIVORS

Witness Justice
National nonprofit organization providing programs and advocacy for survivors of violence and trauma.
P.O. Box 2516
Rockville, MD 20847
1.301.846.9110

IF YOU ARE A VICTIM OF A CRIME

- Don't resist.
- Never pursue your attacker.
- Call the police. Dial 9-1-1 in case of an emergency
- **REPORT CRIME!** Get resources for help.

VICTIM'S RIGHTS

National Center for Victims of Crime
The leading resource and advocacy organization.
2000 M Street NW, Suite 480
Washington, DC 20036
1.202.467.8700
Fax: 1.202.457.8701
http://www.victimsofcrime.org

Office for Victims of Crime
A component of the Office of Justice Programs - US Department of Justice, that provides contact information for victim service providers, victim assistance and financial assistance/compensation programs nationwide, and network of attorneys and allied professionals dedicated to facilitating civil actions brought by crime victims.
ITVERP Resource Center
810 Seventh Street NW, 8th floor
Washington, DC 20531
1.800.363.0441
http://www ojp.gov/ovc

Targets/Weapons

In general summation, **AVOID** depending on weapons such as a gun, knife, pepper spray or other advertised "ultimate self-defense weapon." Unless you really know how to properly use them they can be a false sense of security, forcibly taken away, and used against you. In a moment of panic, do you have time to reach in your purse for a weapon, does the spray nozzle face you when you press the button? Nothing you can buy, or place in your purse, can be more effective than your own natural weapons: **elbows, feet, fingers, hands, and knees**.

First of all, mental preparation and quick-wittedness are your **ALERT** and **AWARE** weapons. Second, natural weapons are simple to use, easy to aim, and can't be taken away from you. If you find it hard to jab an assailant in the eye with your fingers or other object, be prepared to defend. **Remember, whatever you do or use, it is to distract/disorient the attacker long enough for you to run, escape to a safer area.** Never count on one strike to take care of the problem. Follow through with strikes, kicks, blows to the vulnerable areas, such as head, eyes, nose, throat, groin, knees, and shin. Grab a wad of hair and pull him down. Always initiate these tactics with a scream or forcible confident yell.

Be **ALERT** and **AWARE** of other persons near you.

YOUR FIVE TARGETS AND WEAPONS

Eliminate potential dangers by being **ALERT, AWARE,** and recognizing to **AVOID**. Thinking safety with proper mental habits and a cool head are keys, but threats to your personal safety may still occur. **AVOID** denying its existence and your feelings of panic until it is too late are bad habits. For example, if one of your exercises in January was to list five dangerous situations, what ways did you write that could have prevented or **AVOIDED** a crime of burglary or possibly rape? Was it installing proper window locks or using a device that allows windows to be opened only a few inches?

The strategies of recognizing and **AVOIDING** are never complete unless you are always **ALERT** and follow through. Your mindset must always be offensive, not defensive. By taking the offense in a potential attack, you gain the element of surprise and stay aggressive to follow through. If you hesitate, you may lose that element of surprise to strike first, immobilize, and escape. Attack while the attacker still thinks he has the advantage. Any technique becomes worthless if you are unwilling to use it or hesitate because, "I don't want to hurt my attacker," or "I can't hit in the eye or groin." **AVOID** giving the attacker the advantage.

FIVE VULNERABLE TARGETS

Be **ALERT** to never just hurt, but always injure your attacker to immobilize and to escape. If your attacks are not aggressive enough the attacker will be aggravated to counterattack.

1. The **eyes** are the most **vulnerable** area for attack.
2. A **groin** blow can make it impossible for him to stand upright. Can immobile him. Escape.
3. **Knees.** A slight force applied can cause enough pain and/or injury to immobilize for your escape.
4. Strikes to the back of the **neck** or throat areas can be used as follow-through strikes.
5. **Nose** strikes cause blurring of vision.

If, and only if, you know when to attack and know how to attack as a last resort, you already have body weapons to use on several targets of the assailant. Don't take chances by kicking or throwing punches the wrong way. It is not recommended to deliver blows unless you have practiced, learned how to apply, and mastered. Don't risk injuring yourself and making attacker angrier.

WEAPONS

Every attack must have the ingredients of accuracy, force, and speed. Every attack must include follow-through attacks that continue until your attacker is immobilized and you escape to safety.

Fingers and thumbs can injure an attacker by gouging eyes with thumbs and jabbing with the fingers. If you are going to wince, rather than strike or poke out eyes, then it is not a concern to you to protect yourself and/or save your life.

Hands can deliver blows using hand strikes to throat (make thumb form a V with fingers); a heel palm as an upward thrust to jaw, nose, or head (meaty portion); finger jabs using nails to rake or strike eyes; cupping hand and striking the ear hard with slap of palm; a hammer punch to strike the face, collarbone, ear, and groin from behind (rolling fingers tightly into each other, placing thumb against bent fingers and using the side of the fist, not knuckles).

Your **legs** are the **strongest** part of your body, because they establish more leverage, and longer and greater muscle mass to deliver more forceful blows, such as kicking attacks. Use heel of foot, or high heel, to slam down on attacker's foot or scrape shin.

Use the top of your **knee** to deliver strikes to the groin. Step into the kick as if you were kicking a door in.

Your **voice** should be used each time you attack with aggressive, terrifying, loud and long screams as if King Kong just picked you up.

Biting is an excellent defense. Angle your face to apply pressure to sensitive areas such as neck, ear, face, arm, and groin. Use an elbow strike to chin, face, neck, head, and groin from behind (tip of elbow).

IMPROVISED WEAPONS

- **Book or package(s).** Aim the sharpest edge toward the attacker's nose, throat, or under chin.
- **Cup of hot coffee/tea.** Throw in face.
- **Flashlight.** Jab, end first in groin, knees, neck, or nose. Resist swinging it sideways.
- **Heel.** Used like a hammer, while a stiletto heel can be used like a spike.
- **Ink pen/pencil.** Thrust into eyes, throat, face, and hand to cause injury.
- **Keys.** Keys are always available when you return to your car or home and should be held in-between fingers ready to be used as a weapon. Grasp them with the sharp end of each key protruding out and in-between fingers. Jab sensitive areas, such as eyes, ear, nose, and throat.
- **Newspaper/Magazine.** Rolled, they make a good hand weapon to jab into the throat or under the nose. Is not effective for swatting or slapping.

- **Noisemaker.** Compressed air siren, a loud piercing scream and whistle in a short-long-short signal (S.O.S.), if possible.
- **Portfolio/briefcase.** Hard edges against throat or wrist.
- **Purse and contents.** Can be used as a shield against a knife. Use it as a weapon pointing the most rigid portion at the attacker, jabbing under nose or throat. Sharp objects in purses, such as combs, lipstick, brushes, pens, pencils. They may be difficult to get at the last moment, but something to add in your "tool box."
- **Umbrella.** Use as a shield and/or spear. Point sharp end and jab in solar plexus, groin, or throat. If attacker grabs and tries to pull you in, let him and kick hard into his groin or knees (only you know if you can do this).

At Home...

- **Dinner napkin.** Can be used to choke or flick into eye to disorient.
- **Cup of coffee.** Throw in face and/or eyes.
- **Mop or broom.** Thrust into solar plexus, groin, or ribs.
- **Ink pen/pencil.** Thrust into eyes, throat, face, and hand to cause injury.
- **Keys.** Ears, face, eyes, or under the chin.

Prepare. Develop a plan. Visualize. Rehearse.

It is important to mentally rehearse (mindset) as it prepares you to be **ALERT, AWARE** and **AVOID.** You should go over in your head how far you are willing to go and for what reason. Mental rehearsal gives you permission to defend yourself and create a mindset that you will survive and worth defending. Go over your five situations you wrote in January or write some "what if" scenarios and questions. Practice mental imagery or visualization with your strategies.

PEPPER SPRAY

The idea of *The Unique Triple A*™ is to be prepared. When you decide to take pepper spray with you, it is recommended to have it immediately available, such as on your key ring, belt, in hand, especially when walking or jogging alone, entering hallways, elevators, parking lots. After spraying the attacker **across** eyes, escape immediately and call police. Use of pepper sprays in eyes causes severe skin, eye, and respiratory irritation.

TASERS AND STUN GUNS

The advantage is to give you enough time to get safely away from your attacker. DISTRACT and RUN AWAY.

Taser guns work by shooting out two Taser probes roughly fifteen feet apart. They are electronically charged and give a sharp electrical shock that stuns the person, usually for up to 30 seconds, which is not overly long. Use that time to escape quickly and yell for help.

The stun gun is a risk for the user because the tool is only effective at short distances and temporary. Users have to be at arm's length to their aggressor to transmit the charge into the attacker. The major drawbacks comes at the expense of the user who must press the stun gun into an individual for a certain amount of time, or else the charge will not be enough to stop an attacker. The attacker could grab hold of the stun gun itself and turn it on the individual using the stun gun.

STRIKING TOOLS

The Kubotan, typically no more than 5.5 inches in diameter of hard material, is applied as a weapon, pressure point or pain compliance to strike bony, fleshy and sensitive body parts, such as the bridge of the nose, eyes, fingers, forearms, groin, joints, knuckles, neck, ribs, shins, stomach, solar plexus, spine, temple, and wrists. As mentioned earlier, everyday items, such as hairbrushes, pens, and flashlights can be substitutes.

Don't lose time digging in the bottom of your purse or fumbling around to obtain your personal protection items. Keychain adaptable personal protection products can be attached to purses, briefcases, or wallets. Whether you decide to purchase personal protection items to wear on body, key chain or in purse, be prepared for the unexpected. Owners of all tools should familiarize themselves with the weapons or seek assistance through their local law enforcement agency.

CAUTION/WARNING/DISCLAIMER

The use of any of these improvised weapons or devices for any purpose other than self-defense is a crime under law. Illegal use is punishable by imprisonment, fines, or both. Not to be purchased by minors, felons, anyone addicted to narcotics, or where prohibited by law.

Remember, do not solely rely on any self-defense product for protection. **AVOID** dangerous and poorly isolated areas, and use the buddy system when possible. Relying on other weapons rather than being **ALERT, AWARE,** and taking reasonable precautions to **AVOID** situations where self-defense becomes necessary can be a false sense of security.

There are five traditional senses to use in being **ALERT, AWARE, AVOID**: sight, hearing, smell, touch, and taste. The relationships between health, emotions, the senses, and *The Unique Triple A*™ strategies, help make sensible choices.

Questions

A Reading Group Guide...

(A helpful answer guide to questions at end of section).

TEST YOUR KNOWLEDGE

I. Answer all questions True or False in reference to information from this handbook guide.

1. _____ The groin is the most vulnerable area on a man's body.

2. _____ The safest way for a single woman to list name on your mailbox is last name and first initial only.

3. _____ While your neighbors are on vacation, you see a moving van that starts to load their furniture. Your best approach is to have your husband or neighbor request identification.

4. _____ Your defense tactics give you the element of surprise.

5. _____ This handbook is focused on unarmed attacks only.

II. Group Discussion. Assess the "what if's" to the following scenario. What "zone(s)" should you be in?

You are shopping alone at night and returning to your parked car. You feel an uneasy gut feeling and possibly see a shadow nearby, but you brush it off and quickly run to your car with an armful of packages.

THE FOX, CAT, HOUNDS, AND THE HUNTERS
An Aesop Fable

A fox and cat were out walking when the fox began boasting to the cat his clever devices for escaping from any situation.

"I have a whole bag of tricks that contain a hundred ways to escape from my enemies."

"I have only one, but it has always worked for me," said the cat. "I think it is better to have one trick that works than waste time attempting to choose from a hundred that might."

"No, that is just too dumb and not clever enough," said the fox.

Just then, they heard the cries of a pack of hounds growing nearer, and the cat scampered up a tree and hid in the branches.

"That was my one trick, what is yours?" said the cat to the fox.

The fox began to think of one way, then of another, like run, hide, or jump in a burrow. While debating, the hounds came nearer and nearer, and the fox, in his hesitation to find a burrow to fit his body, wasted time. Confused by so many choices, the hounds soon caught him and was killed by the huntsmen.

What is the moral of this story pertaining to *The Unique Triple A*™ safety strategies? What "zone" or "zones" appear?

IV. Driver Practice Test

1. **You may drive off of the paved roadway to pass another vehicle:**

   - ○ If the shoulder is wide enough to accommodate your vehicle
   - ○ If the vehicle ahead of you is turning left
   - ○ Under no circumstances

2. **You are approaching a railroad crossing with no warning devices and are unable to see 400 feet down the tracks in one direction. The speed limit is:**

   - ○ 15 mph
   - ○ 20 mph
   - ○ 25 mph

3. **When parking your vehicle parallel to the curb on a level street:**

   - ○ Your front wheels must be turned toward the street.
   - ○ Your wheels must be within 18 inches of the curb.
   - ○ One of your rear wheels must touch the curb.

V. Book Cover Observation Exercise.

Assess the book cover.

What "zone(s)" are illustrated?

What criminal opportunities do you see on the book cover with the criminal lurking in the background? What opportunities does he see?

How are the female and male subjects' targets for crime?

NOTES:

ANSWER GUIDE

I. True or False. F, T, F, F, T

II. Group Discussion. If you were in a parking lot, hands full of packages, ask yourself where your keys are and/or pepper spray? In your purse? Where is your cell phone? Whistle?

Discuss other options, analysis. Where was potential victim? Was the situation at night? Was the shadow cast because of parking lot lighting or was it in the daytime? What could have **AVOIDED** this situation? Potential victim dressed to attract attention (jewelry, alone), or wearing heels, or carrying more packages than needed to look like a victim? Discuss the Color Codes of **AWARENESS** and where these zones apply to the situation from first encounter to final resolution.

III. Fox, Cat, Hounds, And The Hunters. Your five senses should have been on the **ALERT** in the Yellow Zone and immediately in the Orange Zone when your sense of hearing first heard the cries of the pack of hounds. You switch immediately to Red Zone. It's on and now you are mentally prepared and thinking strategy. You're looking for an avenue of escape and you know what you are going to do, because you practiced *The Unique Triple A*™ and are **ALERT** and **AWARE** to **AVOID** the hounds and the hunters. You imagined all your senses in your mind (hearing, vision, smell), to your environment. You have that one trick or avenue of escape. The purpose of this story exercise means that it takes your mind longer to choose between multiple options than it does to go with just a prepared one. The fewer choices you have, the faster your response.

IV. Driver Practice Test. Under no circumstances, 15 mph, and within 18 inches.

V. Book Cover Observation Exercise.

LEFT SIDE (FEMALE)

- Day crimes as illustrated by sun.
- High hedges hide a criminal. Woman very close to hedges for surprise attack. Not **ALERT, AWARE** to **AVOID**.
- Expensive jewelry (earrings, necklace, ring, watch) attracts attention.
- Hands full of packages.
- Purse with straps across chest. Straps can be pulled over head and/or used to choke or injure woman while she struggles.
- High heels can make it physically difficult to run. Can easily twist ankle/foot.

RIGHT SIDE (MALE)

- Night crime as illustrated by moon.
- Briefcase with straps on shoulder can be easily pulled away. Male victim may struggle for it.
- Expensive watch.
- Close to high hedges.

What else did you observe? Can packages be used as a weapon? Purse? Heels?

These safety guide exercises are suggestions set out to demonstrate the keys to **ALERTNESS, AWARENESS,** and **AVOIDANCE**.

NOTES:

Appendix

CHARTS

HEALTH RECORD SUMMARY

An Ounce of Prevention...

	Blood Pressure	Blood Sugar	Cholesterol	Pulse	Weight
Jan					
Feb					
Mar					
April					
May					
June					
July					
Aug					
Sept					
Oct					
Nov					
Dec					

Track important medical information on a monthly basis in this chart. Before you begin, make copies for ongoing years. After each year has ended, save as an excellent reference source for your health history. Maintain a full medical log and medical records with it. Check with your doctor on required medical exams for your individual health and age.

MEDICATION FLOW SHEET

DATE   MEDICATION/ALLERGIES   **REFILLS**
                                                    Date/Amount

_____

_____

_____

_____

_____

_____

_____

_____

_____

_____

_____

_____

_____

_____

_____

_____

_____

_____

_____

_____

GIFTS RECEIVED

DATE	GIFT RECEIVED	FROM	√ THANK YOU NOTE

EMERGENCY INFORMATION FORM

MAKE COPIES FOR UPDATES
Personal Medical History
(If applicable, do the same for
CHILDREN WITH SPECIAL NEEDS)

Name: _____ Birthdate: _____

Physician: _____

Physician Telephone Numbers: _____

_____

Physician Address: _____

_____

Your Medical Condition:

_____ Medication: _____

_____ Medication: _____

_____ Medication: _____

Allergies: Medications, Foods to be Avoided and Why:

_____

_____

_____

_____

_____

_____

PLEASE CHECK WITH YOUR PHYSICIAN OR VIAL OF LIFE WEB SITE FOR CORRECT FORMS AND INFORMATION.

SUSPECT DESCRIPTION FORM

The following brief guide can aide in criminal identification. Detailed Suspect Description Templates, used by law enforcement for victims and witnesses are easily accessible on law enforcement web sites or law enforcement agencies.

Event Date: _____ Time of Event: _____

Location: _____

Hair: _____ Eyes: _____ Glasses _____

Facial Hair: _____ Scars: _____

Tattoos: _____

Sex: ___ Race: _____ Height: ____Weight:_____

Age: _____ Complexion: _____

Speech/Accent: _____

Hat: _____ Shirt: _____

Jacket/Coat: _____

Pants: _____

Jewelry/Piercings: _____

TIPS TO BE A GOOD WITNESS
Do not jeopardize your safety.
Report immediately to law enforcement.

WEAPON TYPES / SUSPECT VEHICLE

Semi-Auto Revolver

Pump Shotgun   Rifle

2-Door Convertible

4-Door Sedan

Sport Utility

Pick-Up Truck

Van/Mini-Van

Motorcycle

Color: _____

Make: _____

Model: _____

Body Style: _____

Year: _____

License #: _____

Window Tint: _____

No. of Occupants: _____

Rims/Tires: _____

Head/Tail Lights Shape: _____

Dents/Damages: _____

Direction of Travel: _____

SUMMING UP

Now that you've completed a year, I want to thank you for reading my book and thinking about the information provided.

Reading daily affirmations is one thing, but putting its contents in practice is completely different.

Don't be hard on yourself. Practice makes perfect. Let the information percolate and see which affirmations pop out to you that may suggest a vulnerable area or an AHA moment.

Start a journal or write down your thoughts. Review the Test Your Knowledge quizzes. Practice different approaches until you feel comfortable and confident to follow through.

By investing in your safety makes a difference in benefiting yourself, others and your community. You raised **ALERTNESS**, **AWARENSS** and **AVOIDANCE** around a greater mission that can help others empower, equip and educate themselves with hope.

About The Author

Diane Robinson is a retired 35-year police sergeant with teaching experience in crime prevention and *The Unique Triple A*™ to audiences of all ages, men, women, children, seniors, handicapped, and students. It is her desire and mission to be of service in making a difference through quality resources and programs that benefit people and communities.

Diane began training in the martial arts in the mid-1960s, studying under Chuck Norris, earning belts in Taekwondo, and performed stunt work during her law enforcement career. She currently provides dignitary and entertainment protection.

She is an active volunteer member of various Southern California non-profit and civic organizations, including Sisters in Crime, Mystery Writers of America and Children's Book Writers of Los Angeles (CBW-LA). She authored several short stories in CBWs two published Anthology books.

The Los Angeles native is also a descendant of Francisco X. Sepulveda, patriarch of a prominent Spanish-Mexican family in early California. Currently writing the first in a historical murder mystery novel series that follows Francisco in Eighteenth Century Colonial Alta California. Consider Francisco, a Spanish soldier turned investigator Tracker, as a different protagonist with dark secrets, fighting the underworld.

Diane divides her time between Southern California, Canada, and her ranch on a Washington state island. She enjoys beach activities, charity, civic and environmental work, equestrian riding, gourmet cooking, and painting. She is completing a Doctorate in Public Administration.

Diane is currently authoring a series of *The Unique Triple A*™ books, and conducting presentations and workshops on *The Unique Triple A*™ to groups, upon requests.

Did you like Diane's *The Unique Triple A*™ *Safety Handbook?*
Visit her website and learn more at:
http://www.dianerobinsonauthor.com

Turning Inspirations Into Results At
http://www.dianerobinsonauthor.com

*... **books that inspire
and celebrate
remarkable journeys***